Surgical Management of Nasal Obstruction: Facial Plastic Surgery Perspective

Guest Editor

DANIEL G. BECKER, MD

OTOLARYNGOLOGIC CLINICS OF NORTH AMERICA

www.oto.theclinics.com

June 2009 • Volume 42 • Number 3

SAUNDERS an imprint of ELSEVIER, Inc.

W.B. SAUNDERS COMPANY

A Division of Elsevier Inc.

1600 John F. Kennedy Boulevard ● Suite 1800 ● Philadelphia, Pennsylvania 19103-2899

http://www.theclinics.com

OTOLARYNGOLOGIC CLINICS OF NORTH AMERICA Volume 42, Number 3
June 2009 ISSN 0030-6665, ISBN-13: 978-1-4377-0597-3, ISBN-10: 1-4377-0597-9

Editor: Joanne Husovski

Otolaryngologic Clinics of North America (ISSN 0030-6665) is published bimonthly by Elsevier, Inc., 360 Park Avenue South, New York, NY 10010-1710. Months of issue are February, April, June, August, October, and December. Business and Editorial Offices: 1600 John F. Kennedy Blvd., Suite 1800, Philadelphia, PA 19103-2899. Customer Service Office: 6277 Sea Harbor Drive, Orlando, FL 32887-4800. Periodicals postage paid at New York, NY and additional mailing offices. Subscription prices is $264.00 per year (US individuals), $488.00 per year (US institutions), $129.00 per year (US student/resident), $347.00 per year (Canadian individuals), $613.00 per year (Canadian institutions), $390.00 per year (international individuals), $613.00 per year (international institutions), $199.00 per year (international & Canadian student/resident). Foreign air speed delivery is included in all *Clinics'* subscription prices. All prices are subject to change without notice. **POSTMASTER:** Send address changes to *Otolaryngologic Clinics of North America*, Elsevier Periodicals Customer Service, 11830 Westline Industrial Drive, St. Louis, MO 63146. **Customer Service: 1-800-654-2452 (US). From outside the United States, call 1-314-453-7041. Fax: 1-314-453-5170. E-mail: journalscustomerservice-usa@ elsevier.com (for print support) or journalsonlinesupport-usa@elsevier.com (for online support).**

Reprints. For copies of 100 or more of articles in this publication, please contact the Commercial Reprints Department, Elsevier Inc., 360 Park Avenue South, New York, NY 10010-1710. Tel.: 212-633-3812; Fax: 212-462-1935; E-mail: reprints@ elsevier.com.

Otolaryngologic Clinics of North America is also published in Spanish by McGraw-Hill Interamericana Editores S.A., P.O. Box 5-237, 06500 Mexico D.F., Mexico.

Otolaryngologic Clinics of North America is covered in *MEDLINE/PubMed (Index Medicus), Current Contents/Clinical Medicine, Excerpta Medica, BIOSIS, Science Citation Index,* and *ISI/BIOMED.*

Printed and bound in the United Kingdom
Transferred to Digital Print 2011

Contributors

GUEST EDITOR

DANIEL G. BECKER, MD
Clinical Associate Professor, Division of Facial Plastic & Reconstructive Surgery, Department of Otorhinolaryngology, University of Pennsylvania Hospital, Philadelphia, Pennsylvania; Becker Nose and Sinus Center, Sewell, New Jersey

AUTHORS

GREGORY BARKDULL, MD
Surgical Resident, Division of Otolaryngology—Head and Neck Surgery, UCSD School of Medicine, San Diego, California

DANIEL G. BECKER, MD, FACS
Clinical Associate Professor, Division of Facial Plastic and Reconstructive Surgery, Department of Otorhinolaryngology, University of Pennsylvania Hospital, Philadelphia, Pennsylvania; Becker Nose and Sinus Center, Sewell, New Jersey

BENJAMIN S. BLEIER, MD
Resident, Department of Otolaryngology, University of Pennsylvania, Philadelphia, Pennsylvania

JASON D. BLOOM, MD
Resident, Department of Otolaryngology, University of Pennsylvania, Philadelphia, Pennsylvania

MICHAEL A. CARRON, MD
Chief, Division of Facial Plastic and Reconstructive Surgery, Department of Otolaryngology—Head and Neck Surgery, Wayne State University School of Medicine, Detroit, Michigan

MOHAMAD CHAABAN, MD
Staff Physician, Department of Otolaryngology—Head and Neck Surgery, University of Chicago Hospitals, Chicago, Illinois

MINAS CONSTANTINIDES, MD, FACS
Director of Facial Plastic and Reconstructive Surgery, Department of Otolaryngology—Head and Neck Surgery, New York University School of Medicine, New York

CHRISTINA L. COREY, MD
Division of Facial Plastic & Reconstructive Surgery, Department of Otolaryngology—Head and Neck Surgery, Stanford University School of Medicine, Stanford, California

ERIC J. DOBRATZ, MD
Clinical Instructor, Department of Otolaryngology—Head and Neck Surgery, Fellow in Facial Plastic and Reconstructive Surgery, University of Minnesota, Minneapolis, Minnesota

WALEED H. EZZAT, MD
Department of Otolaryngology—Head and Neck Surgery, Thomas Jefferson University, Philadelphia, Pennsylvania

STEPHEN A. GOLDSTEIN, MD, FACS
Assistant Clinical Professor of Otolaryngology, Director, Section of Facial Plastic Surgery, Department of Otolaryngology—Head and Neck Surgery, University of Pennsylvania, Philadelphia, Pennsylvania

DAVID GUDIS, MD
Resident, Department of Otorhinolaryngology, University of Pennsylvania Hospital, Philadelphia, Pennsylvania

SETH E. KAPLAN, MD
Resident, Department of Otolaryngology, Thomas Jefferson University, Philadelphia, Pennsylvania

JASON HAACK, MD
Department of Otolaryngology—Head and Neck Surgery, Division of Facial Plastic and Reconstructive Surgery, The Johns Hopkins University, Baltimore, Maryland

JUDY LEE, MD
Division of Facial Plastic and Reconstructive Surgery, Department of Otolaryngology—Head and Neck Surgery, New York University School of Medicine, New York

PHILIP J. MILLER, MD
Assistant Professor, Division of Facial Plastic and Reconstructive Surgery, Department of Otolaryngology—Head and Neck Surgery, New York University School of Medicine, New York, New York

SAM P. MOST, MD
Director, Division of Facial Plastic & Reconstructive Surgery, Department of Otolaryngology—Head and Neck Surgery, Stanford University School of Medicine, Stanford, California

IRA D. PAPEL, MD
Associate Professor, Department of Otolaryngology—Head and Neck Surgery, Division of Facial Plastic and Reconstructive Surgery, The Johns Hopkins University, Baltimore, Maryland

STEPHEN S. PARK, MD
Professor and Vice Chairman, Department of Otolaryngology—Head and Neck Surgery, Director of the Division of Facial Plastic Surgery, University of Virginia, Charlottesville, Virginia

EDMUND A. PRIBITKIN, MD
Professor, Academic Vice-Chairman, and Program Director, Department of Otolaryngology—Head and Neck Surgery, Thomas Jefferson University, Philadelphia, Pennsylvania

ANIL R. SHAH, MD
Clinical Instructor, Division of Facial Plastic Surgery, Section of Otolaryngology, University of Chicago, Chicago, Illinois; Private Practice, Chicago, Illinois

JONATHAN SYKES, MD, FACS
Professor and Director of Facial Plastic and Reconstructive Surgery, Department of Otolaryngology—Head and Neck Surgery, University of California at Davis Medical Center, Sacramento, California

BOBBY A. TAJUDEEN
Medical Student, Department of Otolaryngology—Head and Neck Surgery, New York University School of Medicine, New York, New York

JAMES R. TATE, MD
Fellow, Facial Plastic and Reconstructive Surgery, Department of Otolaryngology—Head and Neck Surgery, University of California at Davis Medical Center, Sacramento, California

DEBORAH WATSON, MD, FACS
Associate Professor, Program Director, Residency Training Program, Associate Professor, Division of Otolaryngology—Head and Neck Surgery, University of California San Francisco School of Medicine; and Director, Department of Facial Plastic and Reconstructive Surgery; University of California San Francisco School of Medicine, San Diego, California

W. MATTHEW WHITE, MD
Division of Facial Plastic and Reconstructive Surgery, Department of Otolaryngology—Head and Neck Surgery, New York University School of Medicine, New York

EDWIN F. WILLIAMS III, MD
Clinical Professor of Surgery, Williams Center Plastic Surgery Specialists, Latham Facial Plastic and Reconstructive Surgery, Department of Surgery, Division of Otolaryngology—Head and Neck Surgery, Albany Medical Center, Albany, New York

JEFFREY B. WISE, MD
Clinical Assistant Professor, Division of Facial Plastic Surgery, Department of Otolaryngology, New York University School of Medicine, New York, New York; Private Practice, Wayne, New Jersey

CORY C. YEH, MD
Attending Surgeon, Williams Center Plastic Surgery Specialists, Latham, Facial Plastic and Reconstructive Surgery, Department of Surgery, Division of Otolaryngology—Head and Neck Surgery, Albany Medical Center, Albany, New York

DANIEL ZEITLER, MD
Resident, Division of Facial Plastic Surgery, Department of Otolaryngology, New York University School of Medicine, New York, New York

RICHARD A. ZOUMALAN, MD
Resident Physician, Department of Otolaryngology—Head and Neck Surgery, New York University School of Medicine, New York, New York

Contents

Preface   xiii

Daniel G. Becker

Caudal Septal Deviation   427

Jason Haack and Ira D. Papel

> The nasal septum is a structure poorly understood and appreciated by the lay public and the nonotolaryngologist—head and neck surgeon alike. Deviation of the caudal portion of the nasal septum may result in nasal obstruction, a crooked nose, and columellar irregularities. The correction of a severely deviated caudal septum is one of the most difficult challenges of the otolaryngologist and facial plastic surgeon. A variety of options are available for correction of mild, to the most severe, deflections. This condition, as with all challenges in medicine, should not be a one size fits all or one surgery fits all situation. The skilled surgeon should understand the multiple options available for surgical correction and tailor fit the procedure to the deformity.

Classification and Treatment of the Saddle Nose Deformity   437

Edmund A. Pribitkin and Waleed H. Ezzat

> The saddle nose deformity results from a disruption in the nose's integral support mechanisms. Reconstructive surgeons must not only reestablish facial aesthetic contours but also rebuild the nose's structural framework while preserving or restoring nasal function. The causes and the classification of saddle nose deformities are reviewed, and the preferred techniques of correction and reconstruction are illustrated.

Septoplasty Complications: Avoidance and Management   463

Jason D. Bloom, Seth E. Kaplan, Benjamin S. Bleier, and Stephen A. Goldstein

> Nasal obstruction from a deviated septum is one of the more frequent complaints bringing patients into an otolaryngology office. Despite the significant number of septoplasties performed each year, complications after this procedure are relatively uncommon. Most complications result from inadequate surgical planning or poor technique and often can be prevented. Surgeons should discuss these risks with patients before surgery as part of the informed consent process. This article reviews how complications of septoplasty can occur, compromising the functional and aesthetic aspects of a patient's life, and how attention to detail can reduce the risk for these complications. The septoplasty surgeon must be aware of all the possible complications that may arise so as to convey the benefits and risks of surgery effectively to prospective patients.

Surgical Management of the Septal Perforation   483

Deborah Watson and Gregory Barkdull

> Initial management of a septal perforation involves medical intervention, but there are several surgical options available. Deciding to proceed with a surgical repair is dependent on the etiology of the defect, how the symptoms impact the patient, the extent of damage or impending destruction to the nasal support, and the absence of any active disease process. The literature describes several methods for septal perforation repair; each has its technical challenges because of the tenuous nature of the tissues and limited surgical exposure of the area. This article reviews the diagnostic work-up of septal perforations, the medical management, and the surgical treatment options, with emphasis placed on the open rhinoplasty approach.

Surgical and Nonsurgical Treatments of the Nasal Valves   495

Judy Lee, W. Matthew White, and Minas Constantinides

> Nasal obstruction is known to be associated with a major decrease in disease-specific quality of life, and nasal valve dysfunction can play a considerable role in nasal airflow obstruction. Diagnosis and treatment of nasal valve dysfunction requires a thorough understanding of normal anatomy and function as well as pathophysiology of common abnormalities to properly treat the exact source of dysfunction. As the pathophysiology of the nasal valves has become better understood, surgery designed to treat its dysfunction has evolved. Here, we explore the progress we have made in treating the nasal valves, and the deficiencies we still face.

Open Septoplasty: Indications and Treatment   513

Mohamad Chaaban and Anil R. Shah

> Septal deflections have traditionally being addressed by endonasal techniques. Open septoplasty describes using the open rhinoplasty approach to address septal deflections and deficiencies. Accordingly, the authors will highlight the history of open septoplasty, anatomic aspects, diagnosis of septal deflections, and technical nuances in performing open septoplasty. Accordingly, authors will highlight the history of open septoplasty, anatomic aspects, diagnosis of septal deflections, indications and technical nuances in performing open septoplasty.

Congenital Nasal Pyriform Aperture Stenosis   521

James R. Tate and Jonathan Sykes

> Congenital nasal pyriform aperture stenosis is a rare cause of nasal obstruction in the neonate. This condition is caused by a bony overgrowth of the median nasal process of the maxilla. An appropriate workup includes evaluation for associated anomalies and fine-cut CT. Surgical treatment is indicated in patients with respiratory difficulty or poor weight gain.

Septoplasty Pearls 527

Eric J. Dobratz and Stephen S. Park

> Techniques used for the diagnoses and treatment of septal deformity vary according to indications for the procedure and surgeon preference. Septoplasty is commonly performed to treat septal deformity causing nasal airway obstruction. Various preoperative and intraoperative "pearls" that the authors have found to be helpful in treating septal deformity and nasal airway obstruction are discussed.

Cosmetic and Functional Effects of Cephalic Malposition of the Lower Lateral Cartilages: A Facial Plastic Surgical Case Study 539

Cory C. Yeh and Edwin F. Williams III

> Certain anatomic variations of the lower lateral cartilages can predispose patients to nasal obstruction. One particular orientation is the cephalic malposition of the lower lateral cartilages which often results in both cosmetic and functional nasal effects. This article will discuss the pertinent surgical anatomy, diagnosis, the process to identify patients at risk with cephalic malposition of the lower lateral cartilages, pitfalls, and poor surgical changes that result in external nasal valve collapse. Appropriate diagnosis, prevention, and surgical maneuvers to address this will be discussed.

Nasal Reconstruction of the Leprosy Nose Using Costal Cartilage 547

Anil R. Shah, Daniel Zeitler, and Jeffrey B. Wise

> Leprosy is a chronic granulomatous infection of the skin and peripheral nerves that often leads to gross deformation of the nasal skeleton and subsequent formation of a saddle-nose deformity. Reconstruction of the nose following *Mycobacterium leprae* infection has challenged surgeons for centuries. As a result, a number of different techniques have been attempted with varying outcomes. This article describes the case and surgical treatment of a 37-year old female who presented with a subtotal nasoseptal perforation and saddle-nose deformity secondary to previous infection with leprosy. Reconstruction was achieved via an open septorhinoplasty approach using autologous costal cartilage grafts, yielding a successful postoperative result.

A Patient Seeking Aesthetic Revision Rhinoplasty and Correction of Nasal Obstruction 557

Daniel G. Becker, Jason Bloom, and David Gudis

> Thorough evaluation of a patient presenting with nasal obstruction, including nasal endoscopy and a CT scan when indicated, is recommended to guide proper diagnosis and treatment. The rhinoplasty surgeon should be aware of the differential diagnosis of nasal obstruction and should proceed with thorough evaluation or refer the patient for appropriate complete evaluation.

Treatment of Nasal Obstruction in the Posttraumatic Nose   567

Christina L. Corey and Sam P. Most

> The sequelae of trauma to the nose include nasal deformity and nasal ob-
> struction that can have a long-term negative impact on patient quality of
> life. Successful management of posttraumatic nasal obstruction relies on
> a detailed history, careful analysis, and accurate diagnosis. Dividing the
> nose into horizontal thirds assists in preoperative analysis as well as surgi-
> cal treatment. Adequate treatment of posttraumatic nasal obstruction
> must address deflection of the bony nasal pyramid, septal deformities
> (especially caudal or dorsal), turbinate hypertrophy, and incompetence
> of internal and external nasal valves. Treatment must balance the seem-
> ingly disparate goals of re-establishing structure, improving contour and
> esthetics, as well as restoring the nasal airway.

Treatment of Dorsal Deviation   579

Richard A. Zoumalan, Michael A. Carron, Bobby A. Tajudeen,
and Philip J. Miller

> The deviated nasal dorsum is a complex problem with a variety of pro-
> posed solutions. Straightening the deviated nose should be focused on
> maximizing cosmetic outcome while preserving or improving nasal func-
> tion. Deviations can occur in one or a combination of the nasal thirds. A
> simple approach to treatment is to develop a strategy for each third of
> the nose. Tailoring maneuvers to alleviate problems in each specific third
> helps the surgeon deal with deviations in an effective and straightforward
> manner.

Index   587

FORTHCOMING ISSUES

**Radiosurgery and Radiotherapy
for Benign Skull Base Tumors**
Robert Battista, MD, *Guest Editor*

Sialendoscopy and Lithrotripsy
Michael Fritsch, MD, *Guest Editor*

Technical Innovations in Rhinology
Raj Sindwani, MD, *Guest Editor*

RECENT ISSUES

April 2009
**Surgical Management of Nasal Obstruction:
Rhinologic Perspective**
Samuel S. Becker, MD, *Guest Editor*

February 2009
**Palliative Therapy in Otolaryngology–Head
and Neck Surgery**
Kenneth M. Grundfast, MD, FACS,
and Geoffrey P. Dunn, MD, FASC,
Guest Editors

December 2008
**Revision Endocrine Surgery
of the Head and Neck**
David Goldenberg, MD, *Guest Editor*

RELATED INTEREST

Facial Plastic Surgery Clinics, February 2009
Cosmetic Rhinoplasty
Minas Constantinides, MD, *Guest Editor*

THE CLINICS ARE NOW AVAILABLE ONLINE!

Access your subscription at:
www.theclinics.com

Preface

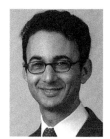

Daniel G. Becker, MD
Guest Editor

Within the specialty field of otorhinolaryngology and head and neck surgery, subspecialties have developed that focus on specific types of problems. We are all familiar with the various subspecialty fields and recognize that there are areas of overlap.

The surgical treatment of nasal obstruction is a large topic. We have divided this into two issues, one with a primarily rhinologic flavor, and this issue with a more facial plastic perspective. Of course, there is overlap; furthermore, we expect that all of the subjects discussed will be familiar to all otorhinolaryngologists.

Nevertheless, otorhinolaryngologists and facial plastic and reconstructive surgeons who have focused their energies on functional and cosmetic septorhinoplasty do offer a unique perspective and experience of the surgical management of nasal obstruction, and this perspective is highlighted in this issue. Many of the articles focus on complex problems related to the septum—treating the caudal septum, a discussion of complications of septal surgery including their avoidance and management, and when to consider the open rhinoplasty approach to septal surgery. Surgical pearls for septoplasty are also considered.

Functional rhinoplasty also naturally receives significant attention in this issue, with consideration of surgical treatment of the saddle nose, treatment of nasal obstruction in the traumatized nose, treatment of dorsal deviation, and surgical and nonsurgical treatment of the nasal valve. Piriform aperture stenosis, a less common form of nasal obstruction, is also considered. A number of facial plastic surgical case studies round out this issue.

I would like to thank the authors whose hard work and contribution to education is acknowledged and greatly appreciated. Also, I would like to thank our publisher

Otolaryngol Clin N Am 42 (2009) xiii–xiv
doi:10.1016/j.otc.2009.03.008
0030-6665/09/$ – see front matter © 2009 Elsevier Inc. All rights reserved.

oto.theclinics.com

and, of course, the reader. We hope that you find the information within this issue useful.

Daniel G. Becker, MD
Division of Facial Plastic & Reconstructive Surgery
Department of Otorhinolaryngology
University of Pennsylvania Hospital
Becker Nose and Sinus Center, LLC
400 Medical Center Drive, Suite B
Sewell, NJ 08080, USA

E-mail address:
beckermailbox@aol.com

Caudal Septal Deviation

Jason Haack, MD, Ira D. Papel, MD*

KEYWORDS
- Deviated nasal septum • Nasal congestion
- Surgical septoplasty • Techniques • Reconstruction

The deviated nasal septum is recognized as a source of nasal obstruction, crusting, epistaxis and recurrent rhinosinusitis. Although the ideal nasal septum would be a straight midline structure in the sagittal plane, most individuals have some degree of curvature or irregularity of the nasal septum. The etiology of a deviated septum is generally congenital, but may also be as a result of trauma or iatrogenic causes. A curved or deviated nasal septum becomes clinically significant when it results in functional or aesthetic morbidity.

Patient quality of life is most often affected when the curvature of the septum results in nasal obstruction. Deviation and obstruction can occur at any point of the bony or cartilaginous septum. Small changes at the dorsal septum can significantly narrow the internal nasal valve, which can further result in dynamic collapse of the upper lateral cartilages. Deflections of the caudal end of the septum result in direct airway obstruction at the nasal vestibule and further congestion caused by tip ptosis and airway collapse.

Aesthetically, nasal septal irregularities can result in twisting of the nose, dorsal humps or depressions, and underprojection. The caudal septum provides a unique set of challenges to the rhinologic surgeon. Unrepaired caudal deviations can cause twisting of the lower third of the nose. Crooked or absent cartilage at the caudal end will also lead to loss of a major tip support mechanism. This can lead to underprojection of the nose and tip ptosis. Finally, the deviated nasal septum can result in columellar irregularities.

Septoplasty, with or without turbinate reduction, is perhaps the most common surgical procedure to address persistent nasal obstruction. Simple submucosal resection of bony or cartilaginous deviations of the midseptum is a technically uncomplicated and highly successful operation. Control of the dorsal septum often requires separation of the upper lateral cartilages and placement of spreader grafts to open and maintain a satisfactory valve angle. It is essential that an appropriate caudal and dorsal strut is left intact to maintain stability of the middle and distal third of the

Department of Otolaryngology, Head and Neck Surgery, Division of Facial Plastic and Reconstructive Surgery, The Johns Hopkins University, Baltimore, MD 21205, USA
* Corresponding author. 1838 Greene Tree Road, Suite 370, Baltimore, MD 21208.
E-mail address: IDPMD@aol.com (I.D. Papel).

Otolaryngol Clin N Am 42 (2009) 427–436
doi:10.1016/j.otc.2009.03.005
0030-6665/09/$ – see front matter © 2009 Elsevier Inc. All rights reserved.

nose. It is commonly accepted that leaving between 1 cm to 1.5 cm is sufficient to maintain support. Loss of this strut, whether through trauma or over-resection can lead to tip instability, valve collapse, and undesired aesthetic alterations of the external nose.

Deflections of the caudal end of the nasal septum are often not addressed at the time of primary septoplasty because of fear of disrupting the caudal strut. By avoiding the caudal strut, the 600 pound elephant in the corner, surgeons are limited in their ability to treat the functional and aesthetic complications of many septal deviations. Satisfactory treatment of the caudal septal deviation requires the surgeon to have a mastery of the complex anatomy of the nasal support structures, an understanding of the options available for treatment, and the ability to execute an appropriate treatment strategy (**Fig. 1**).

ANATOMY

The nasal septum is a bony and cartilaginous structure which separates the nasal cavity into two halves. It also stabilizes the upper and lower lateral cartilages and is a major tip-support mechanism.

The anterior and caudal extent of the septum is cartilaginous. This quadrangular cartilage forms attachments cranially, at the osseous septum, and inferiorly, at the maxillary crest. The maxillary crest terminates anteriorly at the nasal spine. Firm attachments anchor the posterior septal angle of the quadrangular cartilage at this point. A mucoperichondrial flap covers the cartilaginous septum bilaterally, supplying added support and a vascular supply to the underlying cartilage.

Dorsally, the cartilaginous septum is connected to the paired upper lateral cartilages. These cartilaginous structures are fused in the midline and form the internal nasal valve. Caudally, the cartilaginous septum is connected to the lower lateral crura by the intercrural ligament. This fibrous attachment provides additional tip support.[1]

The cranial and posterior septum is primarily osseous. In many patients a small strip of cartilaginous septum extents posteriorly between the perpendicular plate of the ethmoid and vomer.

The perpendicular plate of the ethmoid extends along the posterior and superior extent of the septum in the sagittal plane. Superiorly it attaches to the nasal bones,

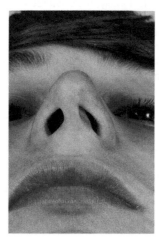

Fig. 1. Caudal septal deviation.

frontal bones and the cribriform plate. Care should be taken when correcting a posterior septal deformity to not disturb the thin attachments to the cribriform plate and risk a CSF leak or injury to the olfactory nerve.

The inferior extent of the osseous septum consists of the vomer. This unpaired bony structure rests on the maxillary crest and forms the midline partition of the nasal choanae (**Fig. 2**).

HISTORY

Attempts to correct nasal septal deformities were described in the medical literature as early as the late 19th century. Early techniques included septal splinting, fracture, and excision. Elaboration of these methods led to excisions that included the vomer, perpendicular plate of the ethmoid, and accompanying mucosa. These techniques were soon abandoned because of the resulting functional and aesthetic morbidity.

Killian and Freer began advocating a more conservative submucous resection at the turn of the century. They emphasized the importance of maintaining the natural mucosal covering as well as leaving a structural strut in place. These early principles have formed the foundation of modern septoplasty.

MEDICAL MANAGEMENT

Medical management of nasal congestion is generally the first line of treatment. Although anatomic abnormalities may exist, hypertrophied nasal mucosa may result in symptoms of nasal obstruction. Treatment with topical nasal steroid sprays can improve airflow and eliminate the need for operative intervention in a minority of patients. The control of inflammatory disease, such as allergic rhinitis or chronic rhinosinusitis, should be maximized before elective septoplasty surgery is recommended.

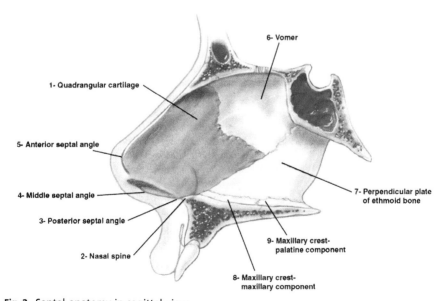

Fig. 2. Septal anatomy in sagittal view.

SURGICAL TREATMENT

Modern surgical septoplasty generally revolves around a few core principles. A submucous approach provides a safe and effective approach to the bony and cartilaginous septum. Care should be taken to identify a precise subperichondrial pocket and maintain this plane of dissection. Surgical resection of the bony and cartilaginous septum may occur without compromising the support and shape of the external nose as long as a 1-cm dorsal and caudal strut is left intact.[2]

The caudal septal deviation can be classified as mild, moderate, and severe. No single method of correction has been shown to be effective in all cases. Most methods of addressing the caudal nasal septum can be classified as either cartilage reshaping procedures or septal reconstruction maneuvers. Although all methods can be approached through either an endonasal or external approach, most caudal septal reconstruction maneuvers are more easily accessible by way of an external approach.

CARTILAGE RESHAPING
Septal Repositioning

Metzenbaum is credited as being the first to address the challenges of the caudal septal deviation. His paper, published in 1929, documents a swinging door method of cartilage repositioning. He describes removing a vertical wedge of cartilage on the convex side of the deformity.[3] The anterior septum is then repositioned in a swinging door like manner and secured.

Many have used modifications of this technique in the last 80 years. Pastorek describes a simple and effective modification of this technique.[4] After excising the vertical wedge of septal cartilage, he repositions the septum to the other side of the anterior septal spine. He describes the use of the septal spine as a doorstop to stop the septum from returning to its native position. Finally, the inferior septum is secured to the spine with a nonresorbable suture.

Translocation of the deviated caudal end to the other side of the anterior septal spine without weakening the caudal septum is an acceptable management strategy in most patients with mild to moderate caudal deviation. A recent paper by Sedwick and Simons describes using this translocation technique with excellent results. Sixty-two patients were retrospectively reviewed from a database of 2043 patients. Access to the septum was achieved by way of a complete transfixion incision and bilateral mucoperichondrial flaps. After a standard septoplasty, the deviated caudal septum was simply repositioned to the midline or contralateral side of the anterior septal spine. After translocation, the caudal end was secured to the septal spine with a polydioxanone (PDS) suture. An inferior strip was removed if the cause of the deviation was excess length. Sedwick reports that 51 of 62 (82%) patients with long-term follow-up reported no postoperative nasal airway obstruction with this technique.[5]

Spreader Grafts

Spreader grafts have been long recognized as a method of opening the internal valve angle and gaining control over the middle nasal vault. Placement of thin grafts between the dorsal septum and upper lateral cartilages will yield consistent and predictable results. Graft material can be obtained from the quadrangular cartilage or perpendicular plate of the ethmoid.

Spreader grafts can also be extended beyond the caudal boarder of the upper lateral cartilages and used to stabilize a deviated caudal septum. Rigid bone, harvested from the ethmoid perpendicular plate, is most often used in this scenario.

The long, thin bone grafts are sculpted to fit holes created for suture placement with an 18 gauge needle. Soft-tissue attachments are released from the caudal septum and the spreader grafts placed. For improved stability it is preferable that the septum be sandwiched between two spreader grafts (**Fig. 3**).[6]

Wedging, Scoring, and Morselizing

Wedging, scoring, and morselizing are generally recognized as one of the most conservative methods of managing the caudal septal deviation. Following the removal of deviated quadrangular cartilage and the preservation of a caudal strut of between 1.5 and 2 cm, the deformed cartilage can be reshaped to create a midline septum. The structure of this cartilage is weakened to allow for reshaping. A series of incomplete incisions are made in the cartilage at the convex surface. The incisions can be made in scoring fashion or serial wedges. Morselizing the caudal cartilage is an alternate method to remove the warped memory of the caudal strut.

Although effective in mild to moderate septal deviations, this method generally should not be selected to manage severe caudal septal deflections. Some authors also question the long-term results and the effect of weakening this tip-support mechanism. These changes after aggressive scoring or moralization may not be apparent for several years. Long-term tip ptosis may result.

Suture Technique

Correction of the curved or bowed caudal septum may also be approached with the use of Mustarde-type sutures. Ellis first described using the same cartilage manipulating techniques that many apply for prominent ears.[7] The convex surface of the deformed cartilage is first scored. Horizontal mattress nonabsorbable sutures are then passed through the cartilage and secured. A series of 2 to 4 Mustarde-type sutures can mold a curved segment of cartilage and establish a more vertical relationship. Although this technique can be effective for mild to moderate deviations, it is rarely effective in the severely deviated nose.

Tongue-in-groove Technique

Stabilization of the repositioned caudal septum can also be done by way of a tongue-in-groove technique. Kridel has published a series of 108 patients using this technique. He describes stabilizing the septum in a groove between the medial crura. Suture is used to secure the septum in this pocket. He reports all patients from his series had satisfactory functional outcomes at follow-up, with no need for revision surgery (**Fig. 4**).[8]

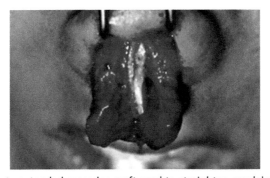

Fig. 3. Ethmoid plate extended spreader graft used to straighten caudal septum.

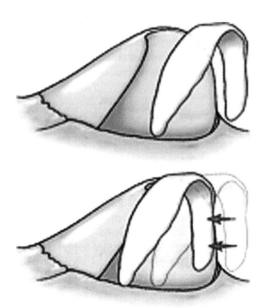

Fig. 4. Tongue-in-groove technique as described by Kridel.

Batten Grafting

Battens are commonly used to stabilize the caudal septum following repositioning, or scoring. Digman first described the use of batten grafting in 1956. Since that time multiple incarnations of this theme have been proposed by various authors.[9–11] Graft material is preferably thin, strong, and of sufficient size to span the length of the septal segment corrected. Authors have described the use of septal cartilage, costal cartilage, ethmoid perpendicular plate, vomer, and calvarial bone.

When employing a batten-graft technique, the deformed caudal end of the septum is first isolated and the region of the defect is identified. The deformed region is then generally weakened by scoring or morselizing to properly reposition the segment. Strips or wedges of cartilage may also be removed to facilitate repositioning. Battens are most often harvested from the posterior septum and carved to fit the desired location. The batten is secured adjacent to the weakened caudal segment to support the tip and prevent recurrence. The batten graft may also be secured to the nasal spine to add additional support.

Alternate sources of grafting material may also be found in the bony ethmoid perpendicular plate or vomer. This region may be accessed when the septum has been depleted because of previous surgery or trauma. Other surgeons prefer this grafting source as a primary modality because of the thin and rigid nature of the bony graft. When using bone for grafting purposes, a series of perforations should be placed with an 18-gauge needle or hand drill before placement. The batten may then be secured in a similar manner with suture to the adjacent caudal septum.

Recent additions to the literature describe the placement of bilateral ethmoid grafts to improved stabilization. Metzinger describes this technique as a "bone sandwich graft." Dyer describes an alternate approach to the batten technique.[12] He describes the complete resection of an isolated segment of caudal septum. He then uses small septal cartilage grafts to recreate the continuity between the caudal and dorsal septum. He likens this technique to that of a titanium miniplate used in a fracture repair and has called it a "cartilage plating graft." Dyer discourages weakening of the remaining caudal septal cartilage or the placement of large grafts overlapping existing segments. A prospective study of 36 subjects treated in this fashion demonstrated a stable airway at 3 to 9 years post-treatment.

Critics of the batten technique point out the addition of cartilage grafts to the existing cartilaginous septum in many cases further narrows an already restricted airway. Others question the long-term viability of the perpendicular plate of ethmoid to stent, and support a caudal septum weakened by morselization.

SEPTAL RECONSTRUCTION

Moderate to severe deviations of the caudal septum may require more aggressive treatment strategies.

Extracorporeal Resection

Complete resection of the cartilaginous septum with reconfiguration of an L-shaped strut has been termed extracorporeal septoplasty. King and Ashley first proposed the principles surrounding extracorporeal septoplasty in 1952.[13] Although first reported as an endonasal technique, most current nasal surgeons use an open approach.

After opening the nose, bilateral mucoperichondrial flaps are raised and the upper lateral cartilages are separated from the dorsal septum. The septum is then disarticulated from the perpendicular plate of the ethmoid, vomer, and maxillary crest regions. The cartilage is removed en bloc and placed in normal saline. The dimensions of the desired strut are identified and the strut is then carved from the straight segments of the previously resected quadrangular cartilage. The graft is then placed in the mucoperichondrial pocket and secured to the dorsal remnant with PDS or permanent suture and at the anterior septal spine (**Fig. 5**).

In the hands of an experienced surgeon, the extracorporeal septoplasty can be used with predictable long-term results for the correction of severe caudal deviations. Gubisch has followed over 2000 patients for the last two decades using the extracorporeal septoplasty with excellent results.[14,15] This series is by far the largest series reported to date.

Complications associated with the extracorporeal technique include the tendency for the development of irregularities of the dorsum postoperatively. Disruption of the keystone area and potential destabilization of the middle third of the nose may occur

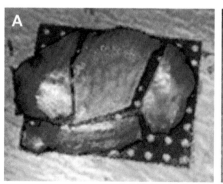 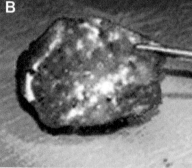

Fig. 5. (*A, B*) PDS foil used to reconstruct extracorporeal septoplasty.

by complete septal cartilage resection. Surgeons note that in some patients notching or saddling of the nose may develop.[16,17]

Alternate techniques of the extracorporeal resection include leaving a portion of the native dorsal septum intact, while resecting the entire anterocaudal septum. This maneuver described by Most[18] maintains the keystone area, while addressing the caudal septum. An anterior septal graft is then formed from a portion of straight cartilage. This graft is then secured at the midline and the remnant dorsal septum. Using this method in a prospective fashion, Most demonstrated an improvement in disease specific quality of life.

CAUDAL SEPTAL RECONSTRUCTION IN THE CARTILAGE DEPLETED NOSE

Although extracorporeal septoplasty is a satisfactory option for reconstruction of the severely deviated caudal septum, the use of native septal cartilage is not an option in many patients. The revision septoplasty patient, or persons who have severe trauma to the nasal septal, will rarely have enough straight cartilage available to reconstruct a satisfactory L-shaped strut. In circumstances when total reconstruction of the caudal end of the nose is necessary, alternate grafting options are available.

Polydioxanone Foil

PDS is a long lasting synthetic polymer commonly used as a suture material. Animal studies have shown complete resorption within 25 weeks.[19] PDS is also available as a semi-rigid foil and can be used as a matrix for septal reconstruction. Gerlinger recently reported a series of 16 subjects in which PDS foil has been used as an extracorporeal template. Smaller pieces of cartilage were sutured to the caudal end of the foil, reconstructing the nasal strut necessary for tip support. Short-term results of the study demonstrated satisfactory improvements in nasal airflow.[20]

Although long-term studies of the use of PDS foil combined with native septal cartilage have not been done, this does seem to be an appealing option for the cartilage depleted patient. If smaller pieces of strong septal cartilage are available, a rigid caudal strut can potentially be reconstructed and temporarily supported with the PDS foil.

Costal Cartilage Reconstruction

Alternate cartilage grafting materials have been used by surgeons for many years. The most popular alternative source in recent years has been costal cartilage. This graft source may be harvested by the experienced surgeon with minimal morbidity. There is ample supply of autologous costal cartilage, and when used as a caudal strut, will easily support the nasal tip. Detractors of the use of costal cartilage cite its unpredictable nature. There is an innate tendency of this cartilage source to warp and further obstruct the nasal airway, leading to unpredictable results. Others cite the possibility of resorption of this grafting material, especially in the caudal region of the nose. Finally, rib grafts may be bulky and difficult to imitate the nature of septal cartilage.

Conchal cartilage is another source of grafting material which is commonly used in the nose. Conchal cartilage is difficult to use as a caudal septal replacement graft because of its curved nature and minimal structural integrity. Authors have described using conchal cartilage sandwiched together in an attempt to reduce its curvature and further reinforce the grafting segment.[21]

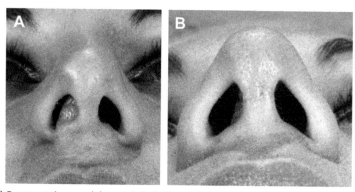

Fig. 6. (*A*) Preoperative caudal septal deviation. (*B*) Correction of caudal septal deviation by translocation over nasal spine.

Nonautologous Materials

Nonautologous materials may also be used for dorsal septal reconstruction; silicone and Medpor are among the long list of possible sources. These materials are easily shaped to fit and tend to be minimally reactive. Difficulties with graft extrusion and implant infection continue to be the biggest challenges facing nonautologous materials.

SUMMARY

The nasal septum is a structure poorly understood and appreciated by the lay public and the nonotolaryngologist—head and neck surgeon alike. This unpaired structure separates the nasal compartments, supports the middle and lower third of the nose, and aids in humidification of airflow. Injury to the septum leads to functional and aesthetic sequelae.

Deviation of the caudal portion of the nasal septum may result in nasal obstruction, a crooked nose, and columellar irregularities. The correction of a severely deviated caudal septum is one of the most difficult challenges of the otolaryngologist and facial plastic surgeon. A variety of options are available for correction of mild, to the most severe, deflections. This condition, as with all challenges in medicine, should not be a one-size-fits-all or one-surgery-fits-all situation. The skilled surgeon should

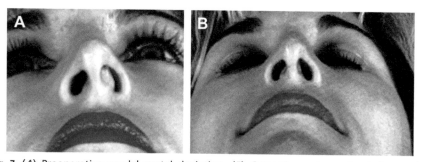

Fig. 7. (*A*) Preoperative caudal septal deviation. (*B*) Correction using extended spreader grafts and suture to nasal spine.

understand the multiple options available for surgical correction and tailor fit the procedure to the deformity (**Fig. 6**A, B), (**Fig. 7**A, B).

REFERENCES

1. Kim DW, Gurney T. Management of naso-septal I-strut deformities. Facial Plast Surg 2006;22:9–27.
2. Gunter JP, Rohrich RJ. Management of the deviated nose. The importance of septal reconstruction. Clin Plast Surg 1988;15:43–55.
3. Metzenbaum M. Replacement of the lower end of the dislocated septal cartilage versus submucous resection of the dislocated end of the septal cartilage. Arch Otolaryngol 1929;9:282–96.
4. Pastorek NJ. Treating the caudal septal deflection. Arch Facial Plast Surg 2000;2: 217–20.
5. Sedwick J, Lopez A, Gajewski B, et al. Caudal septoplasty for treatment of septal deviation. Arch Facial Plast Surg 2005;7:158–62.
6. Metzinger SE, Boyce G, Gigby PL, et al. Ethmoid bone sandwich grafting for caudal septal defects. Arch Otolaryngol Head Neck Surg 1994;120:1121–5.
7. Ellis M. Suture technique for caudal septal devations. Laryngoscope 1980;90: 1510–2.
8. Kridel RW. The tongue-in-groove technique in septorhinoplasty. Arch Facial Plast Surg 1999;1:246–56.
9. Digman RO. Correction of nasal deformities due to defects of the septum. Plast Reconstr Surg 1956;18:291–304.
10. Dupont C, Clutier GE, Prevost Y. Autogenous vomer bone graft for permanent correction of the cartilaginous septal deviations. Plast Reconstr Surg 1966;38: 243–7.
11. Goode RL. Nasal septal surgery. In: Krause CJ, Mangat DS, Pastoreck N, editors. Aesthetic facial surgery. Philadelphia: JB Lipincott Co.; 1991. p. 133–60.
12. Dyer W, Kang J. Correction of severe caudal deflections with a cartilage "plating" rigid fixation graft. Arch Otolaryngol Head Neck Surg 2000;126:973–8.
13. King ED, Ashley FL. The correction of the internally and externally deviated nose. Plast Reconstr Surg 1952;95:672–6.
14. Gubisch W, Constantinescu MA. Refinements in extracorporal septoplasty. Plast Reconstr Surg 1999;104:1131–42.
15. Gubisch W. Extracorporeal septoplasty for the markedly deviated septum. Arch Facial Plast Surg 2005;7:218–26.
16. Gubisch W. The extracorporeal septum plasty: a technique to correct difficult nasal deformities. Plast Reconstr Surg 1995;95:672–82.
17. Mendelsohn M. Straightening the crooked middle third of the nose: using porous polyethylene extended spreader grafts. Arch Facial Plast Surg 2005;7:74–80.
18. Most S. Anterior septal reconstruction. Arch Facial Plast Surg 2006;8:202–7.
19. Boenisch M, Hajas T, Trenite N. Influence of polydionanone foil on growing septal cartilage after surgery in an animal model. Arch Facial Plast Surg 2003;5:316–9.
20. Gerlinger I, Karasz T. Extracorporal septal reconstruction with polydioxanone foil. Clin Otolaryngol 2007;32:462–79.
21. Pirsig W, Kern E, Verse T. Reconstruction of the anterior nasal septum: back to back autogenous ear cartilage graft. Laryngoscope 2004;114:627–38.

Classification and Treatment of the Saddle Nose Deformity

Edmund A. Pribitkin, MD*, Waleed H. Ezzat, MD

KEYWORDS

- Saddle nose • Septal perforation • Implant
- Augmentation rhinoplasty • Graft • Revision • Rhinoplasty

Collapse of the middle vault in relation to the tip and dorsum results in a characteristic saddle nose deformity, which presents significant reconstructive challenges. First recognized in the midnineteenth century as resulting from nasal septal perforations,[1] the saddle nose involves a complex interplay of middle vault support structures (primarily the septum and upper lateral cartilages) and their junctions with the bony dorsum and lower lateral cartilages. Understanding of the pathophysiologic process producing the saddle nose deformity permits effective surgical intervention to reverse the mechanical forces responsible for middle vault collapse and to camouflage its associated cosmetic deformity.

THE STRUCTURAL SUPPORT OF THE NOSE

Nasal structural integrity is maintained by a network of bony and cartilaginous structures connected to each other by dense fibrous tissue and lined internally by a flexible mucoperichondrium. Considered from the viewpoint of a mechanical construction, the nasal foundation or skeletal base consists of the nasal bones, bony septum, pyriform aperture, and the nasal floor. The septal cartilage firmly interlocks with the nasal bones and bony septum to form a "support wall" for the middle vault and the nasal tip. The upper lateral cartilages that make up the "roof" of the middle vault articulate firmly with this support wall and are primarily supported by this wall, although they receive secondary support from their articulations with the nasal bones and lower lateral cartilages. Similarly, despite collaboration from multiple forces as described by Tardy and colleagues,[2,3] nasal tip projection relies ultimately on the septal support wall. Although the inherent strength of the upper lateral cartilages and tip may temporarily prevent collapse of the middle vault or roof, an inherent weakness or injury to the septal support wall results in progressive collapse of the middle vault and deformity of distal tip structures. The roof eventually falls in.

Department of Otolaryngology—Head and Neck Surgery, Thomas Jefferson University, 925 Chestnut Street, 6th Floor, Philadelphia, PA 19107, USA
* Corresponding author.
E-mail address: edmund.pribitkin@jefferson.edu (E.A. Pribitkin).

Otolaryngol Clin N Am 42 (2009) 437–461
doi:10.1016/j.otc.2009.03.004

Critics of this analogy argue that the entirety of this septal cartilage is not necessary to ensure its function. Technically, a door may be placed in a support wall; however, the door must be buttressed on either side and across its top by more substantial columns and beams to ensure structural integrity. Similarly, a 1-cm L-shaped strut of septal cartilage can support the middle vault and tip only if its inherent mechanical properties can resist injury, gravity, and the ravages of time.

The cartilaginous septum's support of the middle vault and tip helps to define the cross-sectional areas critical for adequate nasal breathing. The internal nasal valve bounded by the junction of the upper lateral cartilages with the septum regulates nasal airflow. Accordingly, small changes in this angle result in significant perturbations of airflow.[3] Loss of septal support may also influence the function of the external nasal valve by altering the relationships among the columella, soft triangle, and nasal ala. Progressive weakening of the septal support wall results not only in a cosmetic saddle nose deformity but also in a corresponding loss of nasal function.

DEFINITION

The saddle nose deformity results from a depression caused by a decrease in the structural support of the cartilaginous or bony framework deep to the nasal soft tissue envelope.[4] The septum's articulation with the upper lateral cartilages of the nose and its contribution to tip support through the medial crura of the lower lateral cartilages play an integral part in the cause of the deformity and its correction.[5] Clinicians may use the septal support test[6] to indirectly gauge the strength and stability of the septum by applying force directly to the supratip area. Progressive loss of septal integrity results in a characteristic saddle nose deformity, with depression and splaying of the middle vault, loss of support and overrotation of the tip, decreased vertical projection, retraction of the columella, and widening of the nasal base.[7] Functionally, the internal and external nasal valves are affected, leading to significant difficulties in breathing (**Fig. 1**).

ETIOLOGY

Various pathologic conditions can lead to a saddle nose deformity, but trauma and prior surgical procedures account for most causes in the reported literature.[8–10] Nasal trauma may result in mechanical disruption of the septum or in hematoma formation leading to necrosis of the cartilaginous septum and loss of support.[11] Surgical disruption of septal attachments to the nasal floor, bony septum, and nasal bones, and injudicious resection of the septal cartilage may result in a saddling of the nasal dorsum, although such effects may be delayed for months or years following the procedure.[12] Destruction of the septal mucoperichondrium and subsequent perforation of the septum by prolonged topical use of such vasoconstrictive agents as cocaine and oxymetazoline also commonly result in saddle nose deformities.

Although the cause of a saddle nose deformity may appear evident from the patient's history, a thorough serologic evaluation, CT, and nasal biopsy are required to exclude conditions such as Wegener's granulomatosis, sarcoid, Crohn's disease, and relapsing polychondritis.[13,14] Such illnesses usually result in damage to the septal and middle vault cartilages and involve the bone to a lesser extent.[15] Directed nasal biopsy permits evaluation for neoplastic processes such as inverted papillomas and squamous cell carcinomas in which direct growth of the lesion is locally destructive.[5] Before the popularization of septorhinoplasty, infectious processes were the most frequent cause of saddle nose deformity and included syphilis, leprosy, and septal abscesses.[12,16]

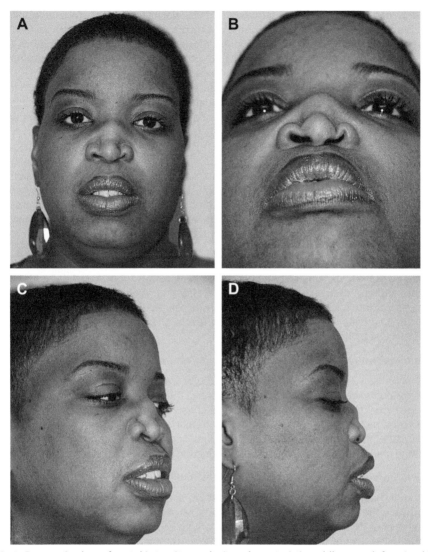

Fig. 1. Progressive loss of septal integrity results in a characteristic saddle nose deformity. (*A*) Depression and splaying of the middle vault. (*B*) Collapse of the internal and external valve with widening of the nasal base. (*C, D*) Decreased vertical projection, overrotation of the tip, and retraction of the columella.

CLASSIFICATION

Numerous classification systems describe the manifestations of a saddle nose deformity. In 1949, Seltzer introduced the system of Joseph, categorizing saddle nose deformities into three types.[5] Type I deformities involved depressions of the middle vault without a loss of the structural support or overlying skin. When a loss of structural support occurred, but no change in nasal length was observed, the deformity was categorized as a type II deformity. Type III deformities required complex reconstructions due to loss of nasal length and support.

Tardy and colleagues[2] also proposed a three-tier classification. Mild deformities included those with a depression of the supratip greater than 1 to 2 mm relative to the tip but no loss of structural integrity. Moderate cases revealed a loss of the quadrangular cartilage, dorsal height, and columellar retraction, whereas severe cases also included major septal deformities and nasal twisting.

Daniel and Brenner[7] introduced a more detailed classification system in 2006 that classified saddle nose deformities into six different types based on clinical findings and pathophysiologic processes. Such a categorization allows a more detailed analysis for reconstructive planning (**Fig. 2**).

Type 0 Deformity: Pseudosaddle

Also termed the pseudosaddle, a type 0 deformity represents a relative depression of the cartilaginous dorsum relative to the bony dorsum. Such depressions may arise naturally or as a result of overresection of the cartilaginous middle vault or overaugmentation of the bony dorsum. Although relatively low, the septal support wall remains solid and the septal support test is always negative (**Fig. 3**).

Type I Deformity: Minor—Cosmetic Concealment

A type I deformity exhibits some minor decrease in septal support, but demonstrates greater supratip depression and columellar retraction. As in a type 0 deformity, the process leading to weakening of the septum has ceased. Augmentation of the dorsum and the columella with soft tissue such as fascia or diced cartilage can effectively restore nasal balance (**Fig. 4**).

Type II Deformity: Moderate—Cartilage Vault Restoration

With progressive weakening of the septal support wall, a type II deformity results. The cartilaginous middle vault begins to collapse and the columella retracts as the nose is "saddled from below." A loss of tip support is concurrently present. Complaints of nasal obstruction secondary to internal nasal valve collapse are common. The reconstruction of the septal support wall and reconstitution of its relationships to the upper and lower lateral cartilage are required to restore nasal valve function and the dorsal contour (**Fig. 5**).

Type III Deformity: Major—Composite Reconstruction

A type III deformity results in obvious flattening and depression of the middle vault. Damage to the septal support wall such as a nasal septal perforation or disarticulation from the nasal foundation drops the septal dorsum and its attached roof, which splays as the upper lateral cartilages are held up only by their articulation with the nasal bones. The nasal tip begins to rotate upward as the columella retrudes and caudal septal support is lost. Reconstruction must first address the loss of integrity by the septal support wall. Following the re-establishment of a stable support wall, the upper lateral and lower lateral cartilages often require further bolstering to maintain the compromised internal and external nasal valve. The dorsal contour can be effectively restored only after this new structure is established (**Fig. 6**).

Type IV Deformity: Structural Reconstruction

A type IV deformity often precludes re-establishment of a normal septal support wall due to a large septal deformity and a concomitant defect in the bony vault. The middle vault is depressed and splayed, altering the configuration of the internal nasal valve. Columellar retrusion coupled with overrotation and deprojection of the nasal tip results in a short nose. The ala are consequently splayed so that the alar base is widened and the external nasal valve is compromised. An associated loss and contracture of the

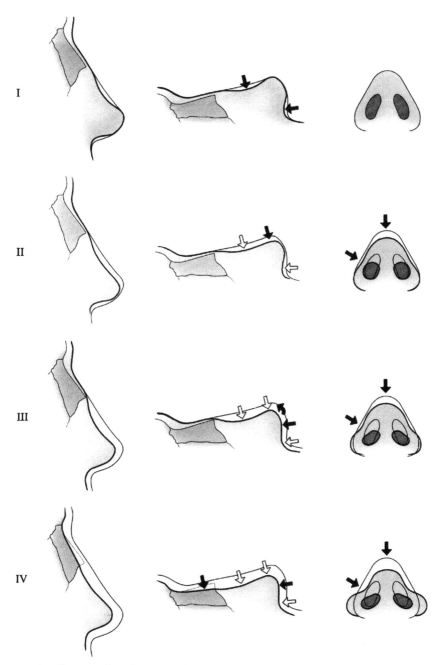

Fig. 2. Classification of saddle nose deformity. Type I has supratip depression and columellar retraction. Type II is more advanced, with loss of tip projection and septal support. Type III has total loss of cartilage vault integrity and flattening of the nasal lobule. Type IV shows progression with involvement of the bony vault. (*From* Daniel RK, Brenner KA. Saddle nose deformity: a new classification and treatment. Facial Plast Surg Clin North Am November 2006;14(4):304; with permisison).

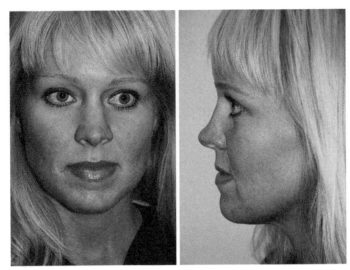

Fig. 3. Type 0 pseudosaddle deformity due to overresection of the cartilaginous middle vault.

nasal lining complicates reconstructive efforts.[7] Functional obstruction results from a multitude of defects including septal perforation, internal valve collapse, external valve collapse, and compromised nasal mucosal function (**Fig. 7**).

Type V Deformity: Catastrophic—Major Reconstrcution

Daniel[6] described type V deformities as "catastrophic" defects requiring total reconstruction of the internal lining of the nose and the bony and cartilaginous nasal vault. Tissues adjacent to the nose are also affected and require attention. Typically, a large flap such as a paramedian forehead flap is required to cover any new framework that is laid down (**Fig. 8**).

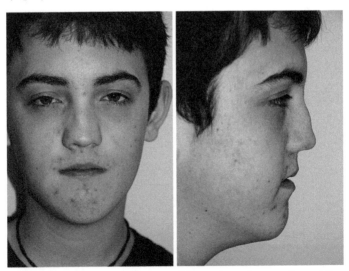

Fig. 4. Type I minor saddle nose deformity exhibits minor decrease in septal support but demonstrates greater supratip depression and columellar retraction.

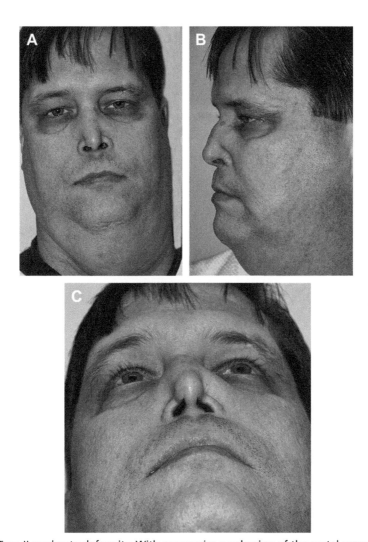

Fig. 5. Type II moderate deformity. With progressive weakening of the septal support wall, the cartilaginous middle vault begins to collapse (A) and tip support diminishes and the columella retracts as the nose is "saddled from below" (B). (C) A loss of tip support and internal nasal valve collapse are common.

RECONSTRUCTIVE MATERIALS
Alloplasts

Nasal augmentation with alloplastic materials such as leather and ivory was advocated as early as the nineteenth century.[1] Ideally, a nontoxic and nonallergenic alloplastic material would be easy to sculpt and sterilize and would resist resorption and rejection.[5] Rigid plastics gave some early hope for alloplastic grafting. They were well tolerated in the body and were nonimmunogenic, but if they became infected, they were subject to extrusion.[17] Furthermore, their hard surface was difficult to mold and gave the nose a hard consistency that could shift with trauma.

Due to their inert biologic properties, silicone implants remain widely used in dorsal augmentation, especially in Asia. A fibrous capsule surrounds these smooth implants

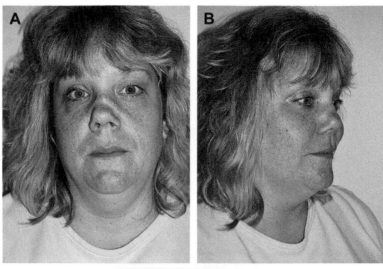

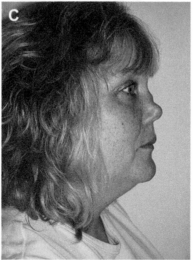

Fig. 6. Type III major deformity. Damage to the septal support wall such as a nasal septal perforation or disarticulation from the nasal foundation results in (*A*) obvious flattening and depression of the middle vault; (*B*) drop in the septal dorsum and its attached roof, which splays as the upper lateral cartilages are held up only by their articulation with the nasal bones; and (*C*) rotation of the nasal tip upward as the columella retrudes and caudal septal support is lost. Reconstruction must first address the loss of integrity by the septal support wall.

that do not integrate with the adjacent tissue and are therefore prone to shifting and buckling (**Fig. 9**).[18] Proponents of these implants refer to their ease of use and, if revision is necessary, their ease of removal. Tham and colleagues[19] retrospectively analyzed 355 patients in which silicone implants were used for nasal augmentation and concluded that silicone was effective, economical, and safe for surgical correction of the Asian nose with its thicker soft tissue envelope. It is unfortunate that follow-up averaged just over 4 months and removal or replacement of the implant was

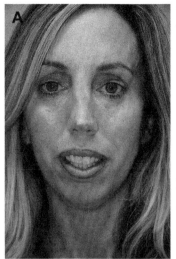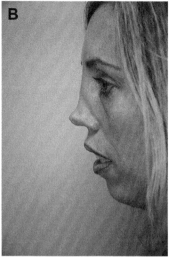

Fig. 7. Type IV deformity involves a large septal deformity and a defect in the bony vault. (*A*) The middle vault is depressed and splayed with a pinched internal nasal valve. (*B*) Columellar retrusion coupled with overrotation and deprojection of the nasal tip results in a short nose.

necessary in 7.8% of patients. Longer-term studies have also reported higher extrusion and infection rates (**Fig. 10**).[20,21]

Expanded polytetrafluoroethylene has been used to fill nasal soft tissue defects and can be effective in camouflaging type 0 and type I deformities (**Fig. 11**). Meticulous material handling, perioperative antibiotic instillation, and long-term follow-up can help limit the relatively high rates of infection, rejection, and fistula formation that have been associated with this material.[22]

A porous high-density polyethylene material that allows ingrowth of connective tissue and more complete integration of the implant into the soft tissue has been studied.[18] A stable, firm surface must be present to permit incorporation, and initial sterile handling of the implant is critical to lower long-term infection risks.[23] Türegün and colleagues[20] reported good cosmetic results with the use of this material implanted into the dorsum of 36 patients over a 3-year period; however, the present authors have noted the susceptibility of the implant to fracture when used as a cantilever-type graft in the reconstruction of larger saddle nose deformities (**Fig. 12**).

Autografts

An autograft uses the patient's own tissue for use in reconstruction. It offers complete tissue immunogenicity and the lowest rates of resorption and extrusion.[24] Donor sites include septal, auricular and rib cartilage, calvaria, and iliac bones. Because of its structural rigidity and easy harvest,[5] septal cartilage is frequently preferred for reconstruction[25] but often cannot be secured in saddle nose deformities without further compromising the integrity of the septal support wall. Conchal and rib cartilage have been reported as secondary candidates.[2,5] Conchal cartilage can be obtained without postsurgical deformity when one maintains the antihelical integrity; however, it lacks structural rigidity.[25] In patients whose ribs have not undergone ossification, rib grafts provide ample rigid cartilage for the fabrication of multiple large reconstructive

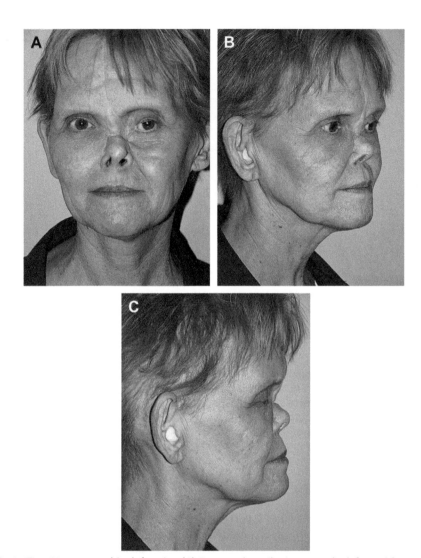

Fig. 8. Type V castastrophic deformity. (*A*) Bony and cartilaginous vault defect with associated orbital and facial deformities. (*B*) Skin contracture and loss of nasal lining compounds extreme nasal shortening. (*C*) Tip cartilage is preserved but deformed by relentless middle and upper vault collapse.

struts.[5] Excess cartilage may also be banked in a postauricular pocket for future use (**Fig. 13**). Nonetheless, donor site morbidity includes the possibility of pneumothorax, postoperative pain, and chest wall or breast deformity.[25]

Numerous techniques have been described for repair of the nasal septal perforations frequently associated with saddle nose deformities. Reconstruction of the nasal septum in three distinct layers using bilateral mucoperichondrial flaps with interpositional grafting has gained widespread acceptance.[26–29] This method consistently demonstrates closure rates greater than 70% and frequently higher than 90% in numerous series. Autologous grafts used for the repair of nasal septal perforations

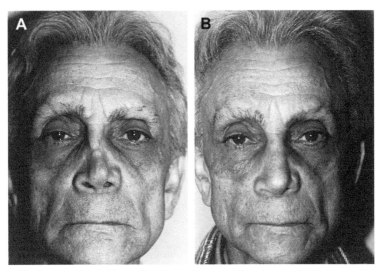

Fig. 9. Buckled and twisted silicone implant (*A*) removed and corrected by way of an open-approach nasal reconstruction with expanded polytetrafluoroethylene dorsal augmentation (*B*).

include temporalis fascia, septal cartilage and bone, pericranium, mastoid bone and perichondrium, tragal cartilage and perichondrium, ethmoid bone, iliac crest, conchal cartilage, and skin grafts.[27,30]

Homografts

A natural human alternative to autografts, homografts are harvested from cadaveric sources. Before harvesting, donors are initially screened for systemic diseases or local infectious processes. The harvested homografts are stored in solution and subjected

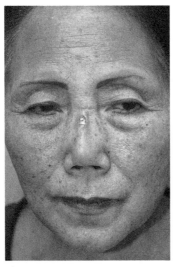

Fig. 10. Extruding silicone implant.

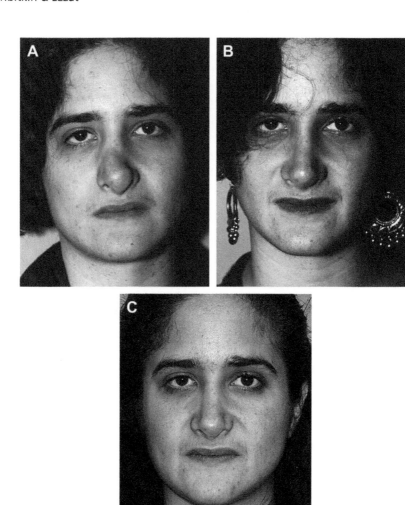

Fig. 11. (*A*) Type I/II deformity resulting from multiple rhinoplasty procedures. (*B*) Restoration of dorsal support with onlay expanded polytetrafluoroethylene grafting (1 year post operation). (*C*) Seven years post operation.

to gamma irradiation at 30,000 to 40,000 Gy to sterilize and reduce the antigenicity of the graft, which allows them to display good tissue compatibility and resist infection.[31] Other benefits include easy availability and the avoidance of donor site morbidity. Gunter and colleagues[32] found no difference in the rate of warping of irradiated cadaveric cartilage versus fresh cadaveric cartilage in vitro over a 4-week period. In both groups, the grafts carved from the periphery of the cartilage tended to warp at a higher rate than those carved from deeper portions of the rib.

The degree of homograft resorption when used in facial reconstruction remains controversial.[33] Early studies demonstrated that the rate of resorption was highly dependent on the area of the face implanted.[34] Kridel and Konior[31] published a series of 122 procedures using irradiated costal cartilage for nasal augmentation. Over an

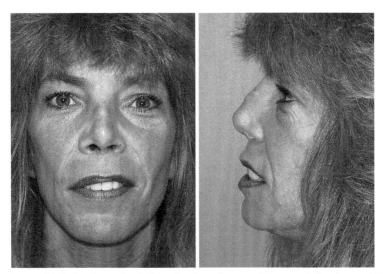

Fig. 12. Porous high-density polyethylene implant fractured 3 years following saddle nose repair.

average follow-up of 15 months, 4 (3.3%) of the homografts showed significant resorption. In 2 of these 4 cases, resorption was attributed to infection from the use of braided suture rather than a natural process. This resorption rate was much lower than that of previously reported studies that failed to specifically address nasal reconstruction exclusively.[33,34]

Noncartilaginous, processed homografts have also become available: an acellular dermal human donor skin tissue matrix can be placed over a stable existing structural framework to augment the nasal dorsum. Although the biocompatibility of the graft is suitable, long-term results have shown a high resorption rate and the need for

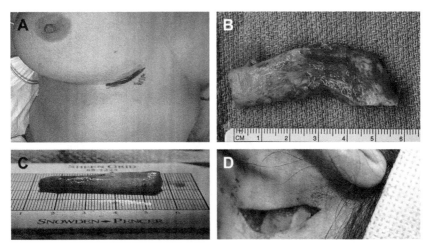

Fig.13. (*A*) Incision for rib autograft. (*B*) Harvested rib autograft. (*C*) Carved rib autograft. (*D*) Excess rib cartilage banked in postauricular pocket.

overcorrection when the graft is used for augemntation.[35] This matrix has been successfully used to repair nasal septal perforations associated with saddle nose deformities.

Xenografts

In general, the use of xenografts harvested from nonhuman sources has met with little success in nasal augmentation. However, the authors previously described the use of porcine small intestinal submucosa [PSIS] as an interposition graft sandwiched between bilateral mucoperichondrial advancement flaps for the successful closure of nasal septal perforations.[36] PSIS is a biologic, acellular, freeze-dried, soft tissue graft that mimics the extracellular matrix environment and encourages angiogenesis, epithelial and connective tissue growth, and differentiation (**Fig. 14**).[36] The greater than 90% closure rate in the authors' 47 patients compares favorably to published results for autografts, with advantages including absence of donor site morbidity, easy graft modification and manipulation, and shorter operative time.

RECONSTRUCTIVE OPTIONS
Type 0 and Type I Deformities

As stated earlier, these types of deformities retain their structural integrity. The septal support wall has been lowered but generally remains strong. Most important, the process leading to the depression of the cartilaginous middle vault relative to the bony dorsum and tip has been arrested. Therefore, the restoration of the dorsal profile may proceed without concern for strengthening or rebuilding the septal support wall.

Injectable filler materials may be employed to correct relative supratip depressions, but lasting corrections generally require the use of onlay and support grafts. As previously described, allografts of silicone and expanded polytetrafluoroethylene may be used successfully but can result in delayed infection and extrusion (see **Fig. 10**). In general, autografts are favored for dorsal augmentation. For example, the use of portions of the alar cartilage as a pedicled flap rotated cephalically and secured

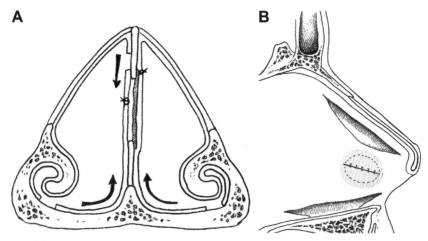

Fig. 14. (A) Axial cross section. PSIS (*yellow*) employed as an interposition graft sandwiched between bilateral mucoperichondrial advancement flaps from the floor of the nose and a unilateral mucoperichondrial advancement flap from the septum. (B) Sagittal cross section.

intraseptally has been reported.[9] Although the investigators stated that this technique offers better correction of the internal nasal valve, dorsum, and projection of the tip, they admitted that overall support is minimal and the technique should be reserved only for minimal supratip depressions. Bare, diced cartilage grafts from the septum, concha, or rib have been used but are associated with the possibility of (1) shifting despite placement in a secure pocket of tissue and (2) palpable irregularities, especially in thinner-skinned individuals.[37] To eliminate these drawbacks, Erol[37] established the method of wrapping diced cartilage in an oxidized cellulose polymer made of polyanhydroglucuronic acid to correct defects of the nasal dorsum, a procedure he named "The Turkish Delight." Other investigators have wrapped inferior turbinate bones in this material for similar corrections.[38] Erol[37] published a series of 2365 patients treated over the course of a 10-year period, with a revision rate secondary to overcorrection and resorption of under 1%.

Daniel and Calvert's[39] attempts to duplicate these results, however, were unsuccessful due to significant resorption noted in all the grafts. When removed, these polymer-wrapped grafts demonstrated a significant foreign body reaction,[40] leading to the resorption of the underlying cartilage. Daniel and Calvert's[39] temporalis fascia–wrapped grafts, however, failed to display a destructive process surrounding the graft, showed minimal evidence of resorption, and retained the regenerative capacity of the cartilage. A smooth contour was attained and no evidence of mobility was observed. These grafts may be inserted into the supratip area through an intercartilaginous incision and do not require overcorrection (**Fig. 15**). Norman[41] described similar success with the use of superficial musculoaponeurotic system fascia with and without the use of cartilage for nasal dorsal correction during concomitant rhytidectomy.

Alternatives to onlay grafts are possible. The upper lateral cartilages may be separated submucosally from the septum and bilateral mucoperichondrial flaps elevated for approximately 1 cm on either side of the dorsal septum. An autologous rib cartilage graft may be fashioned as a triangular wedge and placed as a beam extending from underneath the bony dorsum atop the existing septal cartilage to underneath the cephalic margin of the lower lateral cartilage. The upper lateral cartilage may then be sewn over or to the cartilage beam with 5-0 poldioxane sutures. Horizontal mattress sutures placed through the elevated septal mucoperichondrium and across the junction of the remaining septal cartilage and the rib cartilage beam serve to further secure the construction (**Fig. 16**). Alternately, the remaining cartilaginous dorsum may be hinged at its junction with the nasal bone and advanced on a caudal septal strut or columellar strut to elevate the middle vault (**Fig. 17**).

The columellar retraction noted in some cases of type 0 and type I deformities may be corrected through the judicious use of columellar strut grafts or be camouflaged through the use of filler grafts or materials.

Type II Deformities

In type II deformities, structural reconstruction is required to rebuild the septal support wall and to re-establish the dorsal contour. When present, nasal septal perforations must be corrected though the use of bilateral mucoperichondrial flaps and interpositional grafting. Simultaneous correction of the dorsal profile is possible through the techniques developed by Daniel and colleagues[6,7] and described in the following paragraph.

When the septal support wall has been compromised, a new support beam and column (strut) structure may be fashioned from autologous septal, conchal, or rib cartilage.[2,5] If septal cartilage is to be used, septal support must be maintained by

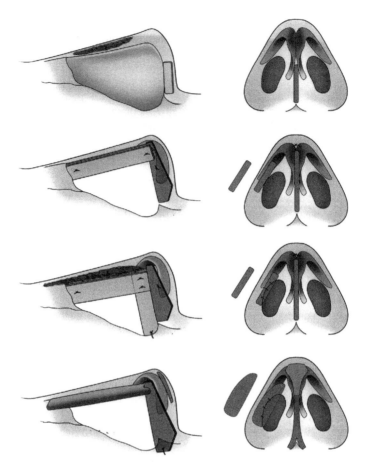

Fig. 15. Treatment of saddle nose deformity. (*Top*) Cosmetic concealment incorporates diced cartilage in the columellar labia angle area. (*Second from top*) A cartilage vault profile restoration with cartilage vault and columellar strut graft. (*Second from bottom*) Composite reconstruction. (*Bottom*) Structural reconstruction. (*From* Daniel RK, Brenner KA. Saddle nose deformity: a new classification and treatment. Facial Plast Surg Clin North Am 2006;14(4):305; with permission.)

harvesting quadrangular cartilage posterior to a line connecting the bony–cartilaginous junction and the nasal spine.[2] Extended vault spreader grafts, consisting of two longitudinal struts of cartilage measuring 20 to 25 mm by 3 mm are placed between the upper lateral cartilages and the septum (see **Fig. 15**) These extended vault grafts form a support beam traversing the septal defect and widen the internal nasal valve to improve breathing. This beam is supported by twin columns: the remaining quadrangular cartilage and bony septum cephalically and a true columellar strut caudally. This caudal strut is placed between the medial crura and rests firmly on the nasal spine, with its maximal width and weight bearing strength at the columellar labial angle.[6] This configuration also provides lobular support and decreases the columellar labial angle.[6] After the desired dorsal profile is obtained, the extended vault grafts are secured to the columellar strut and existing septum by 4-0 and 5-0 polydioxane

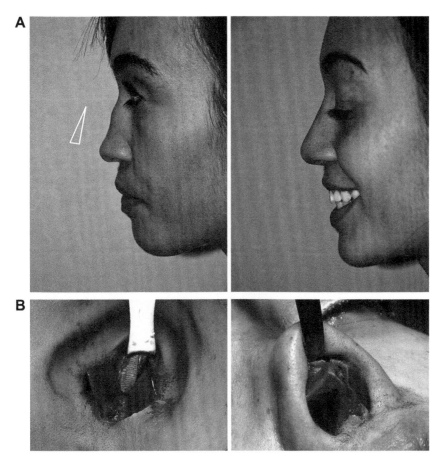

Fig. 16. (*A*) Pre- and postoperative lateral views of type I deformity repaired with a homograft rib triangular wedge augmentation of septum. (*B*) Anteroposterior and oblique intraoperative views. A rib cartilage graft fashioned as a triangular wedge is inserted atop the existing septal cartilage and extends from underneath the bony dorsum to underneath the dome of the lower lateral cartilage. The upper lateral cartilages are sewn to this cartilage beam with 5-0 polydioxane sutues. Horizontal mattress sutures placed through the advanced septal mucoperichondrium and across the junction of the remaining septal cartilage and the implanted cartilage beam further secure the construction.

sutures. The existing upper and lower lateral cartilages may then be attached to this new construction to reconstitute the middle vault and nasal tip.

Type III Deformities

Type III deformities involve extensive loss of integrity by the septal support wall. The dorsal contour can be effectively restored only after a new supporting structure is established. Traditional one-stage approaches involve iliac crest, calvarial, or rib cartilage grafts secured to the bony dorsum and to a dorsocaudal septal/columellar strut (**Fig. 18**). Rib cartilage is obtained from the fifth, sixth, or seventh rib from an incision placed in the inframammary fold in women and directly over the rib to be taken in men as described by Marin and colleagues.[25] For sterility purposes, this rib cartilage is

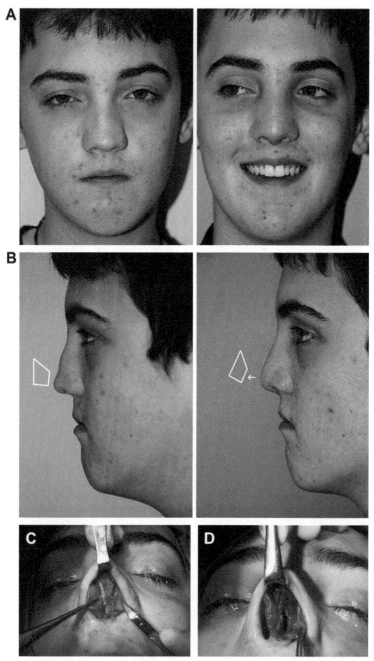

Fig. 17. (*A*) Pre- and postoperative anteroposterior views of type I/II deformity repaired with a hinge advancement of the remaining cartilaginous septum. (*B*) Pre- and postoperative lateral views. (*C*) Septum has collapsed, pulling the upper lateral cartilages down and splaying them. (*D*) Upper lateral cartilages have been divided submucosally from the septum, which has been advanced onto the nasal spine but remains hinged at the bony cartilaginous junction just under the nasal bones.

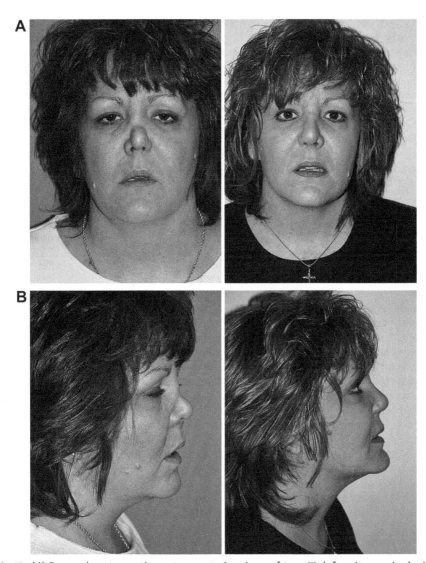

Fig. 18. (A) Pre- and postoperative anteroposterior views of type III deformity repaired with a traditional noncantilevered rib cartilage graft. (B) Pre- and postoperative lateral views.

harvested initially in the procedure, and preliminary carving takes place. Such procedures obviate the need for repair of extensive nasal septal perforations and require less nasal lining than more complex reconstructions. Rib grafts, however, may warp or shift with time under normal nasal stresses.

An alternative composite approach by Daniel[6] involves the re-establishment of a stable support wall through long spreader grafts—described as "pistol" grafts by Gunter and colleagues[42]—carved along the natural curvature of the rib and secured beneath the bony dorsum (see **Fig. 15**). These pistol grafts are secured to a piece of rib cartilage carved to serve as a dorsocaudal septal strut and sutured directly to the nasal spine. The upper lateral cartilages may then be attached to this stable support wall. Adequate nasal lining is critical for the survival of these grafts. Persistent columellar retrusion is addressed through an additional columellar strut. Tip malpositions are corrected by advancing and suturing the medial crura to the columellar strut. When additional projection is required, onlay or shield tip grafts are used.[4] After the structural framework has been established and the tip work completed, dorsal augmentation can proceed as a secondary step. Fascia alone, diced cartilage, or fascia-wrapped diced cartilage grafts may be placed along the dorsum to achieve the desired contour.[7] Lateral nasal wall collapse can be corrected through additional cartilage grafts designed to bolster the compromised internal and external nasal valve. Segments of cartilage as thin as 1 mm can be carved and provide adequate support and aesthetics.[6]

Type IV Deformities

Defects of the bony vault now accompany the complete loss of septal support and contracture of the nasal lining. Composite reconstructions aimed at rebuilding a septal support wall are not possible due to the compromised nasal lining. A new framework for the nose must be fashioned from a cantilevered dorsal graft integrated with a dorsocaudal septal/columellar cartilage strut. Tardy and colleagues[2] reserved the use of autogenous iliac bone crest for reconstruction of these major defects; however, iliac bone harvesting results in significant donor site morbidity and pain.[5] Membranous calvarial bone grafts have been shown to exhibit improved resorption rates over the endochondral bone of the iliac crest. Thomassin and colleagues[43] reported a resorption rate of 13.5% for iliac bone versus 0% for calvarial bone over a mean follow-up of 4 years when correcting moderate and major saddle nose deformities. Calvarial bone has also been used for creation of an L-shaped strut in reconstruction. Such a graft has the advantages of harvesting generous graft material from the same region of the body; direct bone-to-bone contact, improving graft-take rate; and a minimal blood supply requirement.[44] This option is not ideal for patients who have thinning hair, are bald, or have a monocortical calvaria. Iliac crest and calvarial bone grafts address only the central component of the deformity; further harvesting of cartilage is needed for support of the ala and lateral nasal side wall.

A cantilevered osseocartilaginous dorsal graft carved from the ninth rib can also provide adequate structural support and aesthetic contour (**Fig. 19**).[45] Cephalically, this graft is secured to the existing nasal bones with percutaneous Kirschner wires, 1.2-mm titanium lag screws, or a 1.2-mm titanium X-shaped fixation plate. A dorsocaudal septal/columellar strut fashioned from the same rib graft is incised vertically, permitting a tongue-in-groove suture fixation to the dorsal rib graft. This strut is also incised to permit it to straddle the nasal spine. A 4-0 polydioxane suture is passed through a hole drilled through the strut's "legs" and the nasal spine to ensure rigid fixation. Tip projection and lateral nasal wall reconstruction may proceed as described for a type III defect, but results are often limited by extensive contracture of the skin and nasal lining.[4,6,7]

Type V Deformities

The catastrophic loss of nasal support, lining, and skin coverage characterizing the type V deformity requires the use of forehead flaps (**Fig. 20**) or microvascular free flaps to re-establish nasal form and function. Alternately, a nasal prosthetic may be fitted to provide excellent cosmetic camouflage.

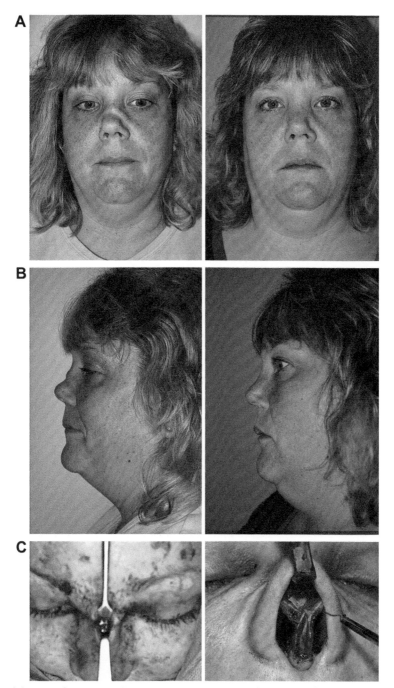

Fig. 19. (*A*) Pre and postoperative anteroposterior views of type IV deformity repaired with a cantilevered rib cartilage graft. (*B*) Pre- and postoperative lateral views. (*C*) Cantilevered dorsocaudal rib graft articulates with a long columellar strut.

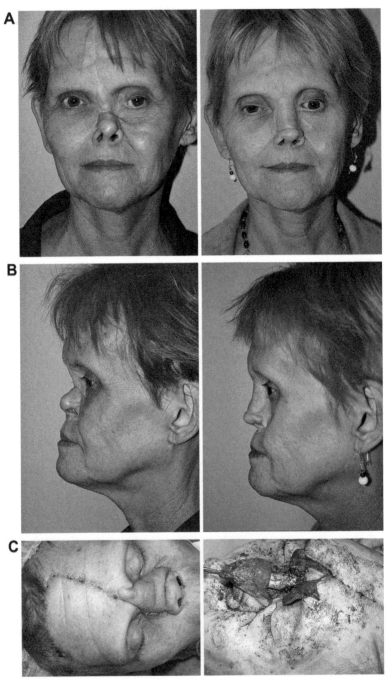

Fig. 20. (*A*) Pre- and postoperative anteroposterior views of type V deformity repaired in two stages. (*B*) Pre- and postoperative lateral views. (*C*) First-stage forehead flap to re-establish nasal lining and skin coverage, followed by cantilevered rib cartilage graft.

SUMMARY

Disruption of the septal support wall results in middle vault depression and widening, columellar retrusion, tip overrotation and deprojection, and nasal shortening that characterize the saddle nose deformity. Over the years, advances in the understanding of nasal mechanics and in autologous grafting techniques have enabled a systematic evaluation and reconstruction of these deformities. A key principle in reconstruction is the re-establishment of a septal support wall through the repair of septal defects or through the creation of a stable column and beam construction. Existing upper and lower lateral cartilages and new cartilage batten, shield, and tip grafts may then be attached to this stable support structure to reconstitute the middle vault and nasal tip, creating a pleasing nasal aesthetic.

REFERENCES

1. Lupo G. The history of aesthetic rhinoplasty: special emphasis on the saddle nose. Aesthetic Plast Surg 1997;21(5):309–27.
2. Tardy ME, Schwartz M, Parras G. Saddle nose deformity: autogenous graft repair. Facial Plast Surg 1989;6(2):121–34.
3. Kim DW, Mau T. Surgical anatomy of the nose. In: Bailey B, Johnson J, Newlands S, editors. 4th edition, Head and neck surgery—otolaryngology, vol. 2. Philadelphia: Lippincott Williams & Wilkins; 2006. p. 2511–32.
4. Emsen IM. New and detailed classification of saddle nose deformities: step-by-step surgical approach using the current techniques for each group. Aesthetic Plast Surg 2008;32(2):274–85.
5. Dyer WK, Beaty MM, Prabhat A. Architectural deficencies of the nose: treatment of the saddle nose and short nose deformities. Otolaryngol Clin North Am 1999; 32(1):89–112.
6. Daniel RK. Rhinoplasty: septal saddle nose deformity and composite reconstruction. Plast Reconstr Surg 2007;119(3):1029–43.
7. Daniel RK, Brenner KA. Saddle nose deformity: a new classification and treatment. Facial Plast Surg Clin North Am 2006;14(4):301–312, vi.
8. Bilen BT, Kilinc H. Reconstruction of saddle nose deformity with three-dimensional costal cartilage graft. J Craniofac Surg 2007;18(3):511–5.
9. Kalogjera L, Bedekovic V, Baudoin, et al. Modified alar swing procedure in saddle nose correction. Aesthetic Plast Surg 2003;27(3):209–12.
10. Yabe T, Muraoka M. Treatment of saddle type nasal fracture using Kirschner wire fixation of nasal septum. Ann Plast Surg 2004;53(1):89–92.
11. Beekhuis GJ. Saddle nose deformity: etiology, prevention, and treatment. Augmentation rhinoplasty with polyamide. Laryngoscope 1974;84:2–42.
12. Andrade M, Fernandes VS, Boleo-Tome JP. Saddle nose: our approach to the problem. Aesthetic Plast Surg 1999;23(6):403–6.
13. Merkonidis C, Verma S, Salam MA. Saddle nose deformity in a patient with Crohn's disease. J Laryngol Otol 2005;119(7):573–6.
14. Shine NP, Hamilton S, McShane DP. Takayasu's arteritis and saddle nose deformity: a new association. J Laryngol Otol 2006;120(1):59–62.
15. Congdon D, Sherris DA, Specks U, et al. Long-term follow-up of repair of external nasal deformities in patients with Wegener's granulomatosis. Laryngoscope 2002;112(4):731–7.
16. Malaviya GN, Husain S. Surgical correction of saddle nose deformity in leprosy—one stage procedure. Acta Leprol 1994;9(2):76–82.

17. Adamson PA. The over-resected nasal dorsum. Facial Plast Surg Clin North Am 1995;3:407–19.
18. Romo T III, Kwak ES. Nasal grafts and implants in revision rhinoplasty. Facial Plast Surg Clin North Am 2006;14(4):373–87.
19. Tham C, Lai YL, Wend CJ, et al. Silicone augmentation rhinoplasty in an oriental population. Ann Plast Surg 2005;54(1):1–5.
20. Türegün M, Sengezer M, Guler M. Reconstruction of saddle nose deformities using porous polyethylene implant. Aesthetic Plast Surg 1998;22(1):38–41.
21. Adams JS. Grafts and implants in nasal and chin augmentation. Otolaryngol Clin North Am 1987;20:913–30.
22. Bracaglia R, Fortunato R, Gentileschi S. Secondary rhinoplasty. Aesthetic Plast Surg 2005;29(4):230–9.
23. Sclafani A, Thomas J, Cox A, et al. Clinical and histologic response of subcutaneous expanded polytetrafluoroethylene (Gore-Tex) and porous high-density polyethylene (Medpor) implants to acute and early infection. Arch Otolaryngol Head Neck Surg 1997;123(3):328–36.
24. Gunter JP, Rohrich RJ. Augmentation rhinoplasty: dorsal onlay grafting using shaped autogenous septal cartilage. Plast Reconstr Surg 1990;86(1):39–45.
25. Marin VP, Landecker A, Gunter JP. Harvesting rib cartilage grafts for secondary rhinoplasty. Plast Reconstr Surg 2008;121(4):1442–8.
26. Goh AY, Hussain SS. Different surgical treatments for nasal septal perforation and their outcomes. J Laryngol Otol 2007;121(5):419–26.
27. Younger R, Blokmanis A. Nasal septal perforations. J Otolaryngol 1985;14(2):125–31.
28. Kridel RW. Septal perforation repair. Otolaryngol Clin North Am 1999;32(4):695–724.
29. Romo T III, Sclafani AP, Falk AN, et al. A graduated approach to the repair of nasal septal perforations. Plast Reconstr Surg 1999;103(1):66–75.
30. Ayshford CA, Shykhon M, Uppal HS, et al. Endoscopic repair of nasal septal perforation with acellular human dermal allograft and an inferior turbinate flap. Clin Otolaryngol Allied Sci 2003;28(1):29–33.
31. Kridel RW, Konior RJ. Irradiated cartilage grafts in the nose: a preliminary report. Arch Otolaryngol Head Neck Surg 1993;119(1):24–31.
32. Gunter JP, Clark CP, Robinson JB. The rate of warping in irradiated and nonirradiated homograft rib cartilage: a controlled comparison and clinical implications. Plast Reconstr Surg 1999;103(1):265–70.
33. Welling DB, Maves MD, Schuller DE, et al. Irradiated homologous cartilage grafts. Long term results. Arch Otolaryngol Head Neck Surg 1988;114(3):291–5.
34. Donald PJ. Cartilage grafting in facial reconstruction with special consideration of irradiated grafts. Laryngoscope 1986;96:786–807.
35. Sclafani AP, Romo T, Jacono AA, et al. Evaluation of acellular dermal graft (AlloDerm) sheet for soft tissue augmentation: a 1-year follow-up of clinical observations and histological findings. Arch Facial Plast Surg 2001;3(2):101–3.
36. Ambro BT, Zimmerman J, Rosenthal M, et al. Nasal septal perforation repair with porcine small intestinal submucosa. Arch Facial Plast Surg 2003;5(6):528–9.
37. Erol OO. The Turkish Delight: a pliable graft for rhinoplasty. Plast Reconstr Surg 2000;105(6):2229–41.
38. Gurlek A, Askar I, Bilen BT, et al. The use of lower turbinate bone grafts in the treatment of saddle nose deformities. Aesthetic Plast Surg 2002;26(6):407–12.
39. Daniel RK, Calvert JW. Diced cartilage grafts in rhinoplasty surgery. Plast Reconstr Surg 2004;113(7):2156–71.

40. Ertas NM, Hucumenoglu S, Bestalti O, et al. The effect of oxidized, regenerated cellulose on diced cartilage xenograft: an experimental study. Ann Plast Surg 2000;45(2):224–5.
41. Norman L. SMAS autografts for the nasal dorsum. Plast Reconstr Surg 1996; 97(6):1249–52.
42. Gunter JP, Rohrich RJ, Adams WP. Special emphasis on dorsal augmentation: autologous rib cartilage. In: Gunter JP, Rohrich RJ, Adams WP, editors. Dallas rhinoplasty: Nasal surgery by the masters. St. Louis (MO): Quality Medical Publishing; 2002. p. 513–27.
43. Thomassin JM, Paris J, Richard-Vitton T. Management and aesthetic results of support grafts in saddle nose surgery. Aesthetic Plast Surg 2001;25(5):332–7.
44. Shipchandler TZ, Chung BJ, Alam DS. Saddle nose deformity reconstruction with a split calvarial bone I-shaped strut. Arch Facial Plast Surg 2008;10(5):305–11.
45. Daniel RK. Rhinoplasty and rib grafts: evolving a flexible operative technique. Plast Reconstr Surg 1994;94(5):596–609.

Septoplasty Complications: Avoidance and Management

Jason D. Bloom, MD[a], Seth E. Kaplan, MD[b], Benjamin S. Bleier, MD[a], Stephen A. Goldstein, MD, FACS[a],*

KEYWORDS

- Septoplasty • Rhinoplasty • Nasal fracture • Septum
- Cartilage • Complications

Although complications after septoplasty are rare, conservative approaches with proper preoperative diagnosis minimize such complications even further. The reported incidence of complications from septoplasty can range anywhere from 5% to 60%.[1,2] Experience, meticulous surgical technique, and comprehensive preoperative planning are all necessary to limit complications. Additionally, the septoplasty surgeon must have a comprehensive understanding of the relevant anatomy, with a specific appreciation for high-risk areas.[3] Although research by Bateman and colleagues[4] has shown that no single surgical maneuver could be identified or associated with an increased risk for septoplasty complications, the need for meticulous surgical technique remains evident. Finally, the importance of experience cannot be understated because it combines methodic and systematic procedure with sound surgical judgment.[3,5]

PREOPERATIVE PLANNING AND EVALUATION FOR SEPTOPLASTY

With any surgical procedure, preoperative planning is essential, and septoplasty is no exception. Nasal obstruction from a deviated septum alone is not always an indication for immediate surgical intervention. Conservative medical therapies should always be attempted and documented before moving forward to the operating room. Significant anatomic obstructions, however, most often still require surgical management.

When evaluating a patient for septoplasty, extensive preoperative assessment is necessary, including a thorough documentation of the patient's past medical and surgical history, allergies, and medications. Two of the more common complications

[a] Department of Otolaryngology—Head and Neck Surgery, University of Pennsylvania, 811 Spruce Street, Philadelphia, PA 19107, USA
[b] Department of Otolaryngology, Thomas Jefferson University, 1020 Walnut Street, Philadelphia, PA 19107-5587, USA
* Corresponding author.
E-mail address: stephen.goldstein@uphs.upenn.edu (S.A. Goldstein).

Otolaryngol Clin N Am 42 (2009) 463–481
doi:10.1016/j.otc.2009.04.011
0030-6665/09/$ – see front matter © 2009 Elsevier Inc. All rights reserved.

from any surgery include bleeding and poor healing. Therefore, it is necessary to review all the patient's preoperative medications, such as anticoagulation and herbal medicines, to reduce these risks. It is also critical to assess the patient's history of tobacco use, because smoking cessation is advised for at least 2 to 4 weeks before and after surgery to avoid delayed nasal wound healing.[1,3] Another consideration in the preoperative workup is a history of intranasal cocaine use. Cocaine users often have abnormalities in the mucoperichondrium leading to decreased vascularity of the septal cartilage secondary to the vasoconstrictive actions of the drug and irritative effects of other contaminating agents. Therefore, this puts these patients at risk for complications during septal surgical procedures.[6]

The presence of significant mucosal disease should raise awareness about several comorbid diseases that may compromise the results of a septoplasty. In fact, any pathologic changes to the septal mucosa on physical examination should arouse suspicion and be evaluated with a biopsy or blood serologies for autoimmune diseases and allergies. The most common changes include chronic inflammation, squamoproliferation, nonnecrotizing granulomas, foreign body giant cells, erosion, and ulceration (**Fig. 1**).[6]

An important step in planning for more complex septorhinoplasty cases includes preoperative photographs.[4] It is crucial to have this confirmation for several reasons, including suitable surgical planning and preparedness, accurate postoperative assessment of aesthetic deformity secondary to the procedure, and protection in the event that litigation is brought about from an unhappy patient.

Finally, as with all procedures, proper informed consent and explanation are important, as is the need to have a thorough discussion of potential complications with the patient. All the following complications, including infection, bleeding, hematoma, septal perforation, scarring, sensory impairment, cerebrospinal fluid (CSF) leak, and aesthetic changes, should be specifically noted, in addition to the necessity of correcting them. The possibilities for revision surgery should also be explained at this time.

ANESTHESIA COMPLICATIONS

Studies have shown that local anesthesia with sedation might lead to fewer complications for patients undergoing septoplasty than general anesthesia. General anesthesia was shown by Fedok and colleagues[7] to require an intervention for bleeding or unintended hospital admission after surgery more frequently. In addition, postoperative

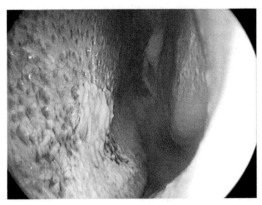

Fig. 1. The anterior septal mucosa reveals chronic inflammation from suspected cocaine use. This inflammation can create a weak or thin mucoperichondrial flap at risk for perforation.

nausea, emesis, and epistaxis rates were higher with general anesthesia, at 36%, 14%, and 3.6%, respectively, compared with local anesthesia with sedation at 8%, 3%, and 0%, respectively. Fedok and colleagues[7] also showed that operating times, in addition to aggregate recovery times, were significantly lower when using local anesthesia with sedation over general anesthesia. When using local or monitored anesthesia care techniques, the authors have found that nasopharyngeal packs are an excellent adjuvant and prevent bleeding into the airway.

The use of topical and injectable anesthetics and vasoconstrictive agents has also been heavily debated, including the use of intraoperative cocaine. Although these drugs have many attractive properties, including rapid onset, prolonged duration of action, vasoconstriction, and decongestant effects, their complications have included mild anxiety, myocardial infarction, cerebral vascular accident, and death. Additionally, there are no present criteria to identify which patients may be at risk for these serious complications.[8] It is important to remember the maximum dosing for each drug. The dose is additive; a 50% toxic dose of two separate drugs may become 100% toxic if they share similar properties. Accordingly, vigilant perioperative patient monitoring with blood pressure, pulse oximetry, and electrocardiography for quick intervention is necessary when using any of these anesthetic medications. Treatment initially includes oxygen, intravenous fluids, and removal of the cocaine-soaked pledgets. If cardiovascular alterations are noted, appropriate anesthesia care is necessary.

FUNCTIONAL COMPLICATIONS

The occurrence of septoplasty complications can be separated temporally. They may be seen at the start of surgery and extend well beyond the completion of the healing phase. Following this time line, the authors review the most common complications.

Hemorrhage: Early

Bleeding or hemorrhage is one of the more common complications of septoplasty, usually occurring during surgery or immediately after surgery. When performing septoplasty surgery, it is important to tell all patients to expect 1 to 2 days of mild oozing after surgery.

True hemorrhage as a result of septoplasty has been reported at a rate of 6% to 13.4%, sometimes requiring admission and overnight observation.[9,10] Acute bleeding during nasal surgery most frequently occurs as a result of poor injection technique or inadvertent mucosal trauma during flap elevation. To prevent bleeding from inadequate injection of local anesthesia, initial topical decongestion with oxymetazoline or cocaine for 5 to 10 minutes before making an incision not only improves visibility but offers the surgeon an opportunity to discern inflammatory mucosal disease from true anatomic septal irregularities. It is beneficial to inject the area in which the incisions are to be made and the important areas of vessel origins (dorsal septum, posterior bony septum, along the nasal floor, and at the anterior nasal spine) adequately. A total of 5 to 6 mL of local anesthesia is typically required for an adequate septal injection when adequate time for vasoconstriction is provided. Proper injections hydrodissect the mucoperichondrium off of the septal cartilage, aiding in flap elevation. In cases of "traumatic" noses or nasal septal fractures, hydrodissection may not work as well and multiple injection sites may help to minimize bleeding.

In terms of traumatic causes of bleeding with septoplasty, in addition to poor technique and accidental mucosal trauma with the septal needle during closure, concomitant intraoperative treatment of turbinate disease is suspected to be the most common cause of postoperative bleeding. The most common source of postoperative bleeding seems to be from the turbinate incision site for inferior turbinectomies. Given their vascularity, it is important to inject the head of each inferior turbinate with approximately 1 mL of local anesthesia 5 to 10 minutes before turbinectomy. Additionally, submucosal resection of the inferior turbinates with a microdebrider is a nice technique that not only allows for a quicker recovery but minimizes mucosal trauma compared with standard turbinate resection followed by cauterization. After the turbinectomy, oxymetazoline-soaked pledgets can be packed against the head of the turbinate for compression to limit bleeding further. They are then removed after extubation to avoid any bleeding at that time. It is always important to secure the pledget strings to avoid accidental aspiration.

There are many methods to prevent significant hemorrhage from occurring after a septoplasty. Although extensive intranasal cautery often tends to lengthen the healing process and the patient's return to normal function, the use of a fibrin sealant may be an acceptable alternative. Fibrin sealant is a formulation based on a concentrate of human clottable proteins and a highly purified human thrombin. The amount of sealant required truly depends on the area of tissue to be treated. Vaiman and colleagues[11] have shown that fibrin sealant, administered by aerosol spray in endonasal surgery, is more effective and convenient than nasal packing. The sealant facilitates hemostasis and prevents or reduces postoperative bleeding and oozing during surgical procedures. Also, as a human blood product, it stimulates normal wound healing of the operated area. No special treatment is required with the use of fibrin sealant, there is no danger of aspiration, and no antibiotics are necessary because there is no foreign object inserted into the nasal cavity. Vaiman and colleagues[11] have shown that postoperative hemorrhage is 22.9% to 25% when using nasal packing and 3.12% to 4.65% when using a fibrin sealant. In fact, Vaiman and colleagues[12] have shown that when using a fibrin sealant during septoplasties, their patients achieved complete resolution of major symptoms; good tissue approximation; and no hematomas, swelling, synechiae, atrophic changes, or adhesions. In contrast, in their group of patients in whom nasal packing was used, 36.5% of patients incurred some level of bleeding and additional discomfort, including sleep disturbance (93%), lacrimation (26%), and pain (47.2%).[11,12]

Finally, it is important to be aware of unusual causes of bleeding from septoplasty. For example, if heavy intraoperative bleeding occurs, it could be secondary to rare occurrences, such as an internal carotid artery-cavernous sinus fistula causing a hyperemic and reactive nose. Be aware of additional signs and symptoms of this complication, including a developing orbital proptosis, deterioration of visual acuity, and pulsating tinnitus.[1]

Cerebrospinal Fluid Leak: Early

Another complication of septoplasty that is exceedingly rare but deserves discussion is CSF leak. This complication is caused by a tear of the dura mater surrounding the brain and its supporting structures of the skull base, which therefore produces a leak of fluid through the formed connection between the subarachnoid space and the nasal cavity. This problem is extremely unusual after septoplasty, but it can be a serious and life-threatening complication if not managed quickly and appropriately. Nasal surgery is the second most common cause of CSF leakage, second only to traumatic skull base fractures. CSF leakage typically occurs early on in the postoperative period, but it may sometimes be days before symptoms develop. Classic presentations include CSF rhinorrhea, headaches, and a salty or metallic postnasal drip.

The literature reports that CSF leakage can occur when elevating the septal mucoperichondrium with a Cottle elevator and tunneling too superiorly on the septum, beyond the limits of the ethmoid roof, or by fracturing the perpendicular lamina, which subsequently can fracture the cribriform plate.[13,14] These areas are at risk because of an intimate connection of dura to a weak and thin bone structure.[13] The anterior cranial fossa is the usual site of this complication, with the roof of the ethmoid sinus and the cribriform plate as the most common sites. CSF leaks in the roof of the frontal and sphenoid sinuses are more likely to occur during endoscopic sinus surgery rather than during septoplasty surgery. When performing a septoplasty and a high bony septal deviation needs to be addressed, a controlled break of the perpendicular plate with a 4-mm chisel or Caplan scissors provides safe separation of the perpendicular plate from the skull base (**Fig. 2**). This is particularly important to remember when re-pairing a nasal septal fracture, especially in the case of a "twisted" nasal septum when the dorsal septum is already malpositioned, likely requiring manipulation.

Early recognition of this complication is important. CSF rhinorrhea may be the first sign. In some cases, if a proper diagnosis is not made, there can be enlargement and remodeling of the bone over time and a dural defect, leading to herniation of the meninges and brain tissue through the defect by pulsation of the brain. This type of skull base defect after septoplasty would subsequently put the patient at risk for an ascending infection. The patients can sometimes present late with the symptoms of meningitis.[13] If septoplasty surgery is performed extremely superiorly in the nasal cavity, avoidance of barometric pressure changes is recommended for 4 weeks after surgery.

The best way to minimize CSF leakage complications after septoplasty is through prevention and early diagnosis. Tawadros and Prahlow[15] have shown that the risk for having a CSF leak after nasal surgery is increased in patients with a low-lying crib-riform plate of the ethmoid roof, specifically found at a level inferior to two thirds of the orbit height on the preoperative CT scan. It is also imperative to prevent this compli-cation with good realization and preoperative awareness of anatomic variations and a less aggressive septoplasty method, especially when manipulating the perpendic-ular plate attached to the ethmoid roof.[14]

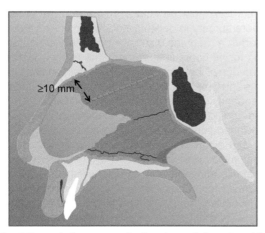

Fig. 2. A controlled cut through the perpendicular plate of the ethmoid reduces torque on the skull base. This should minimize injury to the olfactory groove and cribriform plate. It is important to maintain a 10-mm dorsal strut at the bony cartilaginous junction (seen here). Aiming the chisel or scissors toward the sphenoid sinus should also prevent inadvertent anterior skull base penetration.

If CSF leak has occurred, antibiotics should be given immediately for meningitis prophylaxis. Conservative management of CSF leaks is preferred, with placement of a lumbar drain, reserving surgical repair for patients with a persistent leak despite these therapies. The defect may be approached endoscopically or transcranially to allow for a multilayer repair. If this complication occurs during surgery, it can be repaired endoscopically at that time once informed consent for the additional procedure is obtained.[14] Preoperative informed consent for the septoplasty should include this information, but stopping to inform the patient's family and obtain neurosurgical consultation is recommended. Surgical treatment options for CSF leak repairs include intra- and extracranial approaches, in addition to transcranial approaches, if you need to prevent recurrent meningitis in patients with large defects.[13] Transnasal endoscopic repair is now the standard technique being performed. It is critical to note that meningitis and hydrocephalus can impair the endoscopic correction of a CSF leak and may lead to a poorer surgical outcome.[13]

Infection: Early-Intermediate

As with any surgical procedure, postoperative infection is an important complication to prevent. Overall, there is a 0.48% to 2.5% chance of infection occurring secondary to septoplasty surgery, with infection most likely to occur immediately after surgery.[1,16] Postoperative septoplasty infections are typically localized to the septum and nasal cavity, but they can rarely occur in the form of more dangerous threats, such as meningitis, cerebritis, subdural empyema, brain abscess, and even cavernous sinus thrombosis.[1]

The pathogenesis behind infections after septoplasties stems from the fact that the upper respiratory tract is colonized with many normal bacterial floras. The mucous membranes act as a protective barrier and aid in processing foreign bodies. During septoplasty, those mucous membranes are traumatized and can put the patient at risk for infection and bacteremia by the vascular route within the nasal mucous membranes.[17] There is evidence of transient bacteremia that occurs during open septorhinoplasty. Transient bacteremia is usually harmless in healthy subjects and usually resolves spontaneously without complications; however, the possibility of bacteremia during septoplasty surgery must be kept in mind, and the necessary precautions should be taken before surgery in patients with high risk for cardiovascular infection because this can lead to a dramatic result.[17] Additionally, if septoplasty involves the use of nasal packing for 48 hours after surgery, the risk for bacteremia increases.[18] Even when there is no bony laceration, intracranial infection can occur by direct invasion by way of venous and lymphatic channels of the mucoperiosteal lining of the nasal septum, which is frequently traumatized during septoplasty.[1]

Some patients undergoing septoplasty may be predisposed to infection. It is known that nasal septal deviation impairs mucociliary transport. Septoplasty surgery to fix a deviated septum can significantly improve mucociliary transport; however, the procedure does impair mucociliary transport in the intermediate postoperative stages. Complete recovery of this transport system is established 5 days after surgery if the basal cells and basement membrane of the mucosa remain intact.[19] As noted here, the change in the mucociliary transport system might contribute to an altered nasal mucosal pathogen environment after surgery. Eviatar and colleagues[20] have found that although there is not a major difference in bacterial cultures before and after surgery, as implied by the dominance of *Staphylococcus aureus*, a change in nasal culture results does exist. So, although surgery does not completely disrupt the balance among nasal bacteria, changes in the cultures in the first postoperative month might indicate that the procedure caused mucosal abnormalities secondary to secretions, stasis, crusting, and packing after surgery. These events and circumstances suggest the importance of local environmental factors, aside from growth of bacteria in blood-absorbent packing matrix, in promoting the growth of S aureus.[21]

Although transient bacteremia may occur and be completely asymptomatic, there have been reported cases in which the dangerous systemic toxic shock syndrome has occurred secondary to septoplasty.[21–23] S aureus, considered an important pathogen in the genesis of nosocomial infections, is a frequent cause of bacteremia in postoperative patients.[17] Most physicians credit the nasal packing as the mechanism behind this severe infection. The mechanism is compared with toxic shock syndrome secondary to tampon use on a large mucosal surface.[21,22] When systemic changes, such as fever, diffuse erythroderma and subsequent peripheral desquamation of the hands, hypotension, vomiting, diarrhea, and multisystem complaints with laboratory abnormalities, take place, the patient should be treated promptly, with removal and culture of the nasal packing and hospitalization for the administration of fluids, empiric antistaphylococcal antibiotics, and possibly vasopressor medications.[21,22] This condition warrants early suspicion, recognition, and initiation of appropriate treatment so as to avert significant morbidity and mortality. Given this potential risk and patient discomfort, it may be beneficial to avoid nasal packing unless it is required for uncontrolled bleeding, which is rare.

Septoplasties are considered potentially contaminated operations, but the proportion of patients developing a postoperative infection is small; therefore, perioperative systemic or postoperative antimicrobial prophylaxis is unnecessary.[16] Caniello and colleagues[18] have found that regardless of whether or not antibiotics are used, there is no concerning difference in terms of pain, fever, nausea, vomiting, bleeding, and purulent secretions. In addition, the downside to the indiscriminant use of antibiotics includes severe complications, such as toxic reactions and reduction of the antibody formation stimuli, in addition to representing high costs and encouraging less strict compliance with good surgical practice.[18] The senior author (SAG) regularly provides preoperative antibiotic prophylaxis before induction for all patients undergoing septoplasty. Postoperative antibiotics are given only to those patients who have structural grafting or some type of splint or packing placed. In this situation, 3 to 5 days of treatment should be sufficient.

Again, as with any surgical procedure, there are some circumstances in which antibiotics are necessary. Patients with significant comorbid immune-related conditions, such as diabetes or compromised immunity, may receive prophylactic antibiotics. After surgery, in cases of acute or chronic infection of the operative site, use of cartilage grafts, implantation of allogenic materials, presence of a hematoma, mechanical blockage attributable to nasal packing, or postoperative nasal obstruction producing rhinosinusitis, antibiotics should be administered.[1,16]

Septal Hematoma or Abscess: Intermediate

If unrecognized and not treated, septal hematoma is a significant complication of septoplasty. A septal hematoma may arise in the dead space created between the mucoperichondrial flaps when the cartilage or bony septum is removed during septoplasty. This space is susceptible to accumulation of blood products and the formation of a septal hematoma.[24] The hematoma that forms after surgery can itself lead to several other complications, including ischemia and necrosis of the septal cartilage, decreased septal support, and impaired nasal function. A septal hematoma may also subsequently lead to the formation of a septal abscess, with Staphylococcus, Haemophilus influenza, and, rarely, Pseudomonas being the most common pathogens (**Fig. 3**).[1]

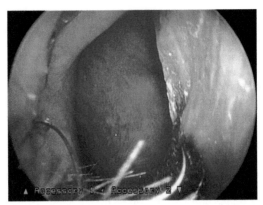

Fig. 3. A septal abscess is seen after septoplasty. It is bulging into the right nasal cavity causing complete nasal obstruction on that side. This complication must be drained immediately to prevent further destruction of the remaining septal cartilage.

To treat a septal hematoma, one must first be able to make the diagnosis effectively. Often, a septal hematoma can be confused with significant postoperative hemorrhage. One way to differentiate between the two entities, other than direct intranasal visualization, is the time of occurrence. A septal hematoma most often occurs during the final phases of surgery and does not appear until the packs or splints are removed.[1]

One method of prevention is the replacement of nasal packing with a continuous mattress or interrupted septal suturing technique. According to Lee and Vukovic,[25] this technique reduces the possibility of a septal hematoma by providing a fine closure, closing any inadvertent tears in the septal mucosa in addition to giving support to the cartilage pieces retained after the septoplasty and keeping them in optimal position. In addition, it reduces patient discomfort by eliminating the need for nasal packing. These are considerations that may outweigh the minor increase in operating time that it takes to perform the suture. Hari and colleagues[24] agree that the use of transseptal sutures obviates the need for packing after surgery. These researchers promote an endoscopic septal suturing technique using a curved needle that they have shown is a more precise method than using a straight septal Keith needle, reducing the risk for accidental needle trauma to the turbinates. Additionally, by placing the knot in the vestibular skin, these researchers have demonstrated a reduction in the risk for intranasal granulation tissue formation. Given this information, however, the senior author (SAG) uses a shorter 11-mm septal Keith needle and closes the mucosal flaps starting anterior to the nasal valve, working along the dorsum and moving posteriorly back to the anterior head of the middle turbinates. The aid of loupes avoids the additional equipment setup. The endoscope is certainly helpful if the middle turbinates are being medialized with the suture in concomitant sinus or concha bullosa surgery. It is important to ensure adequate tension along the suture if there is still slight convexity of the septum. A mild curvature is better treated first with scoring techniques, structural grafting, or additional techniques as opposed to relying on the suture. The position and redraping of the mucoperichondrial flaps is also paramount for balanced healing. The suture knots are removed at 7 to 14 days to minimize crusting and to avoid minor bleeding or irritation. Septal stitches that are supporting grafts are maintained for 2 weeks to allow for resolution of nasal edema. One must be certain not to tighten septal sutures excessively because this may prolong edema and possibly cause septal necrosis.

Should a septal abscess develop, it should be drained immediately. This is most often done first with needle aspiration and then by reopening the septal incision, allowing the abscess to drain. Bilateral nasal packing should then be placed to eliminate septal dead space and prevent fluid reaccumulation. If grafts were used during the operation, they should be removed at that time, if they have become separated. Delayed reconstruction of completely reabsorbed septal cartilage after an untreated septal hematoma or abscess is necessary to prevent septal deformity and further complications. This is done using septal bone, ear cartilage, or even specially prepared allogenic human costal cartilage.[9] Antibiotics should be given after surgery and drainage to prevent further infection and abscess reformation.[1]

Overcorrected Septum: Early or Late

Because of its inherent nature and its underlying structure, septal cartilage is highly unpredictable when disturbed. At the basic level, septal cartilage is a system of interwoven fibers under stress. The stress on the right side of the nasal septum balances the stress on the left side of the nasal septum. Combined, this stress provides equilibrium, allowing the cartilage to remain straight and not curl toward one particular side or the other. Should this equilibrium of stress be disturbed because of injury or surgery, the cartilage could curl or bend away from the weakened side.

Many techniques exist to alter or stabilize septal cartilage. Alterations in the cartilage may range from simple crosshatching of the concave surface to release the surface tension or more aggressive techniques that include partial or full thickness slicing or fracturing of the cartilage, with or without removing the pieces. When full thickness cuts are employed maintaining one mucoperichondrial flap aids the stabilization.[26] Structural grafting provides long term support while internal or external splinting can stabilize the nose during the early phase of healing. For example, one of these techniques uses microcuts in the cartilaginous surface, which can cause stress disequilibrium on the cartilage and may put the septum at risk for secondary curling.[1] One way to correct for this is to reinforce the weakened septum with a Mustarde stitch[27] followed with or without structural grafts. Autogenous cartilage grafts or bone from the posterior septum is used for this purpose because both form a support for the natural septum and have a better chance to endure compared with other implants.[1] Another way to prevent overcorrection of the septum is to provide septal fixation once the intraoperative reconstruction is complete. Fixation can be performed intraseptally, intranasally with packs and or splints, externally by taping through the use of mattress sutures through all layers of the caudal septum, or with a combination of these techniques. Schwab and Pirsig[1] have stated that because of the unpredictability of septal cartilage, none of these techniques always achieves the desired results. The unpredictability, in part, comes from "the memory effect" of cartilage. This is not well understood, but it essentially accounts for the warping of the cartilage back to the preoperative state after septoplasty. This represents one of the reasons why recurrent deformities and deviations can occur. Unfortunately, this is a circumstance that is not always under the control of the surgeon.[9] Given that this is a problem with septoplasty that can be out of the surgeon's hands, it should be explained in layman's terms and included as part of the informed consent process. This problem probably accounts for many of the revision septoplasties that are performed (**Fig. 4**).

To account for this septal unpredictability, many surgeons have compensated clinically by overcorrecting the septum. This complication of septoplasty particularly affects younger patients because they are at higher risk. The incidence of septal overcorrection overall is 2.0%, whereas the incidence for patients younger than the age of 20 years is 7.3%.[28] It is theorized that the need for overcorrection in younger patients

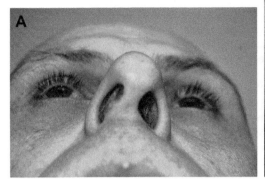
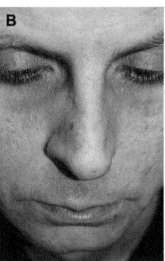

Fig. 4. These photographs demonstrate a postoperative caudal deflection that occurred 2 weeks after the patient's septoplasty. His nose also reveals a nasal pyramid asymmetry that was not addressed at the time of primary surgery.

is related to the growing quadrangular cartilage. According to Lee and colleagues,[28] the central quadrangular cartilage has a high level of metabolic activity, cell replication, and proliferative capacity, all of which decline with age. The anterior free end of the cartilage, however, retains high levels of these aspects throughout the aging process. When overcorrection does occur, it usually presents with symptoms of nasal obstruction on the opposite side of the initial deviation, at least 1 month after the operation is performed.

Septal Perforation: Late

Septoplasty or nasal surgery is the second leading cause of septal perforation after trauma. It is usually a late complication of septoplasty, with an occurrence rate reported between less than 1% and as high as 6.7% (**Fig. 5**).[1,2,5,9,29,30] This complication

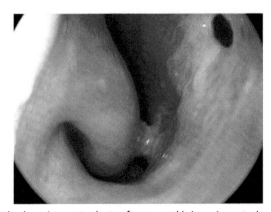

Fig. 5. This patient had a prior septoplasty after a nasal injury. An anterior septal perforation with an additional synechial band is seen at the level of the inferior turbinate.

usually arises as a result of bilateral mucosal tears in corresponding areas on the septum. The symptoms of septal perforation include nasal obstruction, crusting, dryness of the mucosa, intermittent epistaxis, nasal discharge, rhinorrhea, abnormal airflow, whistling during inspiratory nasal breathing, headache, and local pain. Most perforations are small and anterior, interfering with the humidification of inspired air. Larger perforations can lead to other nasal problems, such as atrophic rhinitis. Some perforations may even continue to enlarge and then compromise the structural support mechanisms of the nose, causing a saddle nose deformity.[31] That being stated, most septal perforations are asymptomatic, especially if they occur in the posterior cartilaginous septum. It has been reported that 62% of patients with septal perforations do not experience any symptoms at all.[9,30–32]

Prevention has been found to be the best way to avoid this complication. Otolaryngologists or nasal surgeons need to have a keen awareness of their dissection during septoplasty. Gentle elevation of the mucoperichondrial and mucoperiosteal flaps, especially at the junction of the septal cartilage, vomer, and perpendicular plate of the ethmoid, can help to prevent septal perforation.[2] A common error in nasal septal surgery is the inadvertent dissection in a supraperichondrial submucosal plane (**Fig. 6**), thus leading to perichondrial or periosteal resection and only leaving behind mucosa.[31]

As Kim and colleagues[31] have discovered, the perichondrial layer imparts most of the biomechanical strength to the septal lining. Lining flaps containing perichondrium and mucosa are stronger then flaps with perichondrium or mucosa alone. Dissection in the subperichondrial plane during septal surgery provides a stronger septal flap and may prevent the development of nasal septal perforation during septoplasty and other nasal surgery.

Any intraoperative perforations should be repaired immediately. Simple interrupted 5.0 chromic sutures are placed endoscopically at the time of injury to aid in mucosal healing and prevent perforations. Tears occur mostly over convexities, spurs, or crests, and the resulting surplus of mucosa facilitates endonasal sutures without tension.[9] Vertical tears may be worse than horizontal tears because the septal vessels tend to run forward in an oblique fashion.[2] Additionally, tight suturing of the tears with the use of septal splints and nasal packing should be avoided because septal necrosis can occur.

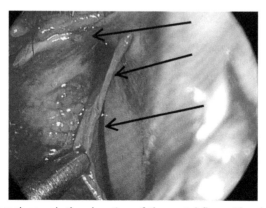

Fig. 6. This photograph reveals the elevation of the septal flap with subperichondrial and submucosal layers. The surgeon needs to stay underneath the perichondrial layer to maintain flap integrity. Submucosal side of mucosal flap (*top arrow*); perichondrial flap (*middle arrow*); subpreichondrial plane above septum (*bottom arrow*).

When septal perforations occur, they should first be managed conservatively with observation and improved nasal hygiene, such as humidification. Even placement of a silastic septal button is a simple procedure to help lessen patient symptoms. If a patient is still experiencing symptoms, a delayed repair can be an option. Closure is usually necessary to alleviate breathing problems, bleeding, crusting, frontal headaches, and nasal whistling. A residual posterior septal deflection of the septum is often present and may also require treatment. It is critical not to destabilize the nose when attempting this repair. It is important to correct these defects because perforations do have a tendency to enlarge slowly over time. Patients often exacerbate the problem and enlarge the size of the perforation from repeated trauma and picking at the crusting that occurs. Again, ample humidification mitigates the intranasal crusting, hopefully avoiding some of these issues.

Bilateral bipedicled mucosal flaps with autogenous grafts seem to be the method of choice for closure of small- to medium-sized (<20 mm) nasoseptal perforations.[30] Closure using this method has resulted in a 90% closure rate and significant improvement in patients' symptoms.[32] Similar results utilizing acellular dermis or porcine small intestine sub-mucosa grafts have also been reported.[33,34] Depending on the type of perforation, a unilateral flap might be more advantageous. The advantages include the fact that it is less invasive and it limits the septal donor area to one side. Additionally, an open or external rhinoplasty approach is sometimes useful because it may facilitate the placement of large connective tissue or homologous grafts to replace the septal cartilage defect.[32] This method is extremely helpful for exposure, especially in helping to close larger (>20 mm) septal perforations.

Adhesions or Synechiae: Late

Adhesions, also known as synechiae, are inflamed bands of adherent mucosa that may cause postoperative nasal obstruction after septoplasty or other sinonasal operations. They are especially common spanning opposing surfaces of abraded or injured mucosa in the nose, most commonly occurring between the septum and inferior or middle turbinates (see **Fig. 5**). They are a common complication of septoplasty, occurring in approximately 7% of patients.[2] Adhesions occur during the late wound-healing phases of recovery. The patient usually remains asymptomatic if the adhesions occur posterior enough; however, patients may complain of postoperative disturbances, attributable to adhesions, from the change in the direction of their nasal airflow.[9] Additionally, not only do adhesions occur intranasally but intercartilaginous incisions for a septorhinoplasty may cause internal nasal valve synechia and result in nasal obstruction from internal nasal valve scarring and narrowing.

Like most complications of septoplasty, the best way to decrease the formation of adhesions is to prevent them. Adhesion formation is best avoided by controlling postoperative infection and minimizing trauma at the time of surgery. There is a great deal of debate in the otolaryngology community about the proper way to prevent adhesions and maintain support of the septum after surgery. Many reports have been published with differing views on the most appropriate method. Here, the authors compare the three most common.

Endonasal applied splints are commonly used to stabilize the reconstructed septum and to prevent the formation of synechia.[1,9] They are usually made of silastic sheeting, and they are left in place for approximately 1 to 2 weeks after surgery. The senior author (SAG) tends to use thin 0.5-mm silicone sheets along the septum if there is significant mucosal trauma or Reuter type splints if the mucosal injury is close to the internal nasal valve and valve support is needed. Although septal splints have been shown to protect against synechiae, there are many disadvantages to using these splints. There seems to be a considerable increase in morbidity when using nasal splints because they can cause a significant increase in pain and discomfort after surgery, especially at the 1-week mark. As a result of nasal splinting, there is a high frequency of drip pad changes related to an increased sanguinous nasal drainage anteriorly and frequent episodes of emesis, potentially indicative of increased posterior drainage, both of which contribute to patient discomfort.[35–37] Interestingly, Malki and colleagues[35] have shown that there is no significant difference in the incidence of adhesions between splinted and nonsplinted patient groups and that if the aim is to prevent adhesions, nasal splints are not justified. Therefore, many surgeons argue that there are no clear advantages to inserting intranasal splints and they should be used sparingly, if at all.[37]

The level of discomfort that patients were experiencing with nasal splinting for long periods led otolaryngologists to employ the use of nasal packing. Usually, nasal packing is used for 4 to 7 days; however, studies have shown that 1 day of intranasal packing is exceedingly preferable to that of 2 or more days because of less patient discomfort and increased cost-effectiveness without an increase in complications.[38] In a study by Schwab and Pirsig,[1] patients with nasal packing were less likely to develop recurrent septal deviation and synechiae and were more likely to have an improvement in the nasal airway, namely, 96% of the patients in the nasal packing group and 64% in the group without nasal packing. Guyuron and Vaughan[36] have shown that when using nasal splints, 60% of patients exhibit discomfort, compared with 22% of patients with nasal packing. Additionally, recurrent septal deviation occurred in 25% of patients who were splinted, as opposed to 23% of those who were packed. Despite the data supporting nasal packing over splinting, in terms of recurrent septal deviation, the role of the septal splint has been relegated to selected cases in which support for the reconstructed nasal septum is necessary.[35]

Although it may seem that most doctors would choose nasal packing as a quick and easy way to support the septum, there are still drawbacks to using this as well. Nasal packing can cause injury to the nares, septum, and nasal mucosa. The packing can dislodge, leading to a risk for aspiration. Long-standing nasal obstruction from packing can lead to nose bleeds, and if the packing remains in place and the patient is not taking antibiotics, it can lead to further infections of the nose, sinuses, and middle ear.[1] Yildirim and colleagues[39] considered the complications related to nasal packing and pointed to the fact that nasal packing after septoplasty causes significant eustachian tube dysfunction, reduction in P_{O_2}, and elevation in P_{CO_2}. The more recent use of septal sutures avoids this gas exchange abnormality, and this same group now believes that it should be the preferred method of nasal septal stabilization as an alternative to intranasal packing. The advantages of septal suturing include the elimination of discomfort for the patients, minimal complications, and septal support outcomes that are almost the same as with nasal packing. When septal suturing is used, there is also a reported shorter hospital stay after septoplasty.[40]

Finally, companies are currently working on products to make septoplasty easier and improve septal support after surgery. Septal staplers are currently in early development; however, long-term studies and cost-benefit ratios are still needed.

Sensory Disturbances: Early-Late

Other complications of septoplasty, and often the most disturbing to the patient, involve the risk for sensory disturbances. These complications include anosmia, palatal sensory impairment, gustatory rhinorrhea, and even blindness.

Anosmia or hyposmia occurs in approximately 1% of patients undergoing septoplasty, with total anosmia on long-term follow-up occurring at a rate of 0.3% to

2.9%.[1,5,9] Transient anosmia can be attributable to nasal packing, clotted blood or crusting, and mucosal edema in the immediate postoperative period. Postoperative anosmia is most likely associated with viral infection, scarring of the ethmoid region, or rare injury to small fibers of the olfactory nerve.[1,9] Although there is little in the way of preventing this occurrence, it is important to understand when this dysfunction occurs. Preoperative testing of olfaction is necessary for comparison with the postoperative state. Should there be any preoperative olfactory disorder, whether temporary or permanent, it should be documented and drawn to the patient's attention.[41]

Some level of sensory disturbance to the anterior palate and central incisors has been reported in 2.8% of patients after septal surgery.[42] This is most likely a result of nasopalatine nerve injury and seems to be secondary to chiseling of the maxillary crest. Conservative resection along the maxillary crest is therefore recommended. Chandra and colleagues[42] also believe that there is a relation between this complication and the use of monopolar suction cautery. To that extent, electrocautery should be avoided near the incisive foramen to minimize this complication. It could be advantageous to make use of bone wax to control blood loss first and to only resort to cautery if necessary.

Guyuron and colleagues[43] have also reported on seven patients with gustatory rhinorrhea after septoplasty. These patients experienced a profuse flow of thin clear nasal drainage on mastication. These researchers postulate that similar to the palatal sensory disturbance, this may be caused by inadvertent injury to the nasopalatine nerve within the septal layers after removal of the deviated portion of the vomer and the perpendicular plate of the ethmoid bone. These patients were treated with antihistamines, which proved to be helpful in these cases.

Additionally, the loss of vision is a rare and frightening complication of septoplasty. The pathogenesis of blindness after a septoplasty may not always be the same, and it may actually arise by means of a variety of mechanisms. One mechanism relates this complication to the use of high-pressure intra-arterial injections of local anesthetics and vasoconstrictors. When these solutions are injected into the membranous part of the caudal septum or into the turbinates, retrograde flow of the injected substances can get into the branches of the ophthalmic artery. These substances can lead to embolism and subsequent occlusion of the feeding vessels of the ophthalmic artery, causing unilateral blindness. Schwab and Pirsig[1] and Monteiro therefore postulate that the loss of visual acuity is best prevented by injecting anesthetic solution (<10 mL) and by avoiding multiple injection sites to reduce the risk of intra-arterial injection. The authors additionally recommend a slower injection to lower the pressure of the injection.

Although rare, direct trauma during septoplasty is another mechanism that has been reported to have caused blindness. While performing a septoplasty, an instrument used to fracture the bony part of the septum may be placed too high and too laterally in the posterior nasal cavity, reaching the area of the optic canal.[44] Again, the importance of recognition and diagnosis of these complications cannot be understated.

AESTHETIC COMPLICATIONS
Deformities after Septal Surgery

The risk for aesthetic complications after septoplasty has specifically been reported as between 4% and 8%.[9] Of these aesthetic complications, there is a 21% to 39.5% risk for a minor aesthetic change and a 1% to 4.5% risk for a major aesthetic change.[4,5,27] There are three major types of septal deformities that may occur secondary to septoplasty. The deformities include aesthetic changes in tip projection, supratip depression or dorsal saddling, and columellar retraction. In some cases, more than one of these complications can occur at a once, and the deformities are often inter-related. According to Daudia and colleagues,[27] the incidence of a minor change (≤ 2 mm) in tip projection is 22.5% and the incidence of a major change (≥ 3 mm) is 3.5%. The incidence of minor saddling is 2.7%, and that of major saddling is 0%. The incidence of minor columellar retraction is 15.4%, and that of major retraction is 0%. Interestingly, Vuyk and Langenhuijsen[4] have shown that there is no relation between general surgical risk factors for septoplasty and the possibility of aesthetic deformity after the procedure. Additionally, there is no increased risk for aesthetic complications in patients who have had previous septal surgery, a frequent situation for patients undergoing septoplasty.

Generally, these aesthetic nasal deformities can occur secondary to a loss of support, cartilaginous mobilization, weakening, and partial resection. For example, after a partial septal resection, if the patient is left with a short dorsal strut, which is now mobile and not properly fixated, the anterior septal angle could counterrotate downward and inward, leading to all three of the previously mentioned deformities.

It is important to keep in mind that although many of the complications of septo-plasty happen during surgery, there are a few of these complications that may occur during the recovery period. For example, deformities can occur secondary to scarring between the columellar skin and mucoperichondrial septal flap, with subsequent inward contraction of the columella and nasal vestibule.[4] Scarring has been shown to be less prevalent when incisions are made over underlying cartilage, as witnessed with a hemitransfixion incision. Poorly designed incisions or inadequate closure tech-nique can lead to entrapment of epithelium into the suture line from the nasal vestibule or lining mucosa. Additionally, scar formation can occur secondary to excessive cauterization of the nasal mucosa. Therefore, the surgeon must be cautious when using this tool to prevent tissue necrosis from the cautery.[1]

Saddle Nose and the Widened Nasal Base

Saddle nose deformity is caused by septal instability and inadequate dorsal cartilage support. The K area, or keystone, is a critical area in which the septal cartilage, paired nasal bones, perpendicular plate of the ethmoid, and upper lateral cartilages meet. When the K-area is disturbed, it can act as a pivot point for the cartilage, leading to the downward and inward rotation of the anterior septal cartilage. This direction of rotation also may cause a subsequently widened nasal base.[9]

A saddle nose deformity is of particular concern among children. As Schwab and Pirsig[1] have pointed out, the introduction of septal trauma or surgery can inhibit the growth of the child's nasal cartilage early in life, and although the septum is fixed in childhood, it can develop into a saddle deformity after puberty. Again, this is partially attributable to the mechanical and biochemical properties of the damaged nasal cartilage.

Saddle nose deformity can be prevented with appropriate septal stability. One way to accomplish this is by keeping the mucosa attached on one side of the septum when tunneling and raising mucoperichondrial flaps. This provides adequate support and preserves the fibers to the premaxillary wing and the anterior nasal spine.[9] Addition-ally, if septal cartilage is resected to remove a septal deviation or for grafting purposes, it is important to maintain a 1-cm "L-shaped" strut of cartilage along the nasal dorsum and caudal septum to prevent dorsal collapse. Another way to prevent this complica-tion is by making sure that the junction between the septal cartilage and perpendicular plate of the ethmoid bone remains intact and impervious to mobilization. As a precau-tion, remember to check the mobility of the caudal septum and fix it with a Wright suture into the nasal spine if it lacks stability. A dislocated septal cartilage can be re-positioned with a guide suture through the columella. This is done with a figure-of-eight stitch to avoid lateral displacement of the caudal septum.[9] At the conclusion of the case, gentle palpation of the dorsum and tip support should be standard. If subtle weakness is present, additional techniques should be performed before waking the patient.

Fig. 7 reveals a patient who had a deviated septum corrected with a trans sphe-noidal hypophysectomy approach for a pituitary adenoma. One month after surgery, she developed a dorsal cellulitis that cleared quickly with a course of antibiotics. No evidence of sinus disease was seen on endoscopy in the sphenoethmoid recess. As her nose healed, left nasal obstruction occurred. Her midvault and internal valves collapsed. These were repaired with a small butterfly graft 6 months after the infection resolved.

Loss of Tip Projection

A loss of tip projection can arise when there is resection of the septum at the attach-ment point to the perpendicular plate or resection of the basal strip of septal cartilage. With these two areas of cartilage resected, mobilization of the septum can take place, effectively leading to ventral nasal collapse.[4] Essentially, in this example, the caudal septum is not appropriately fixated to the anterior nasal spine, leading to a drooping nasal dorsum and sometimes to columellar retraction. Additionally, there is an increased risk for nasal vault collapse and nasal obstruction in patients who have short nasal bones with long upper lateral cartilages.[3]

One way to prevent this problem from occurring is to drill a groove into the premax-illa. This groove can be used to stabilize the septum in place and provide improved fixation.[1] Other ways to correct for loss of nasal tip projection include such techniques as columellar strut grafts, dome-binding sutures, extended columellar strut-tip grafts, caudal extension grafts, premaxillary grafting, shield-like tip grafts, and various onlay tip grafts.[3]

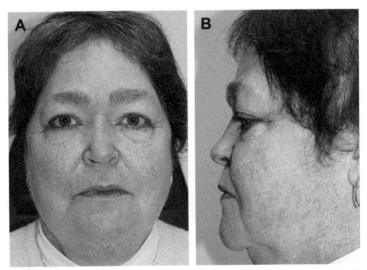

Fig. 7. (*A*) Anteroposterior view seen 4 months after surgery with slight concavity in the mid-dorsum. (*B*) Left lateral view reveals mild 1- to 2-mm midvault collapse causing internal valve collapse.

Columella Retraction

Columella retraction can also transpire in the same manner by which a loss of tip projection occurs. Cartilage resection without proper dorsal and caudal cartilaginous struts or reconstruction causes instability and mobilization at the K-area pivot point.[1]

This deformity can also occur secondary to scar contracture, pulling the remaining septal strut in a ventral and cephalic direction, causing supratip saddling and columellar retraction in addition to possible loss of nasal tip projection. For this reason, it is important to allow 3 to 9 months to pass before evaluating for deformity.[4] Just like the previously listed aesthetic complications of septoplasty, a proper septal reconstruction technique that provides stability for the septum is the only way to prevent this from occurring. In addition, as stated previously, cautious surgical skill that minimizes trauma and scarring is essential.

SUMMARY

Complications after septoplasty can profoundly compromise a patient's functional and aesthetic outcome. The problems associated with septoplasty can lead the nasal airway to obstruct from a loss of support or as a result of the contractile forces of scarring. Incomplete resection, inadvertent nasal trauma, or even overcorrection of the septum may be at fault. It is therefore important for every nasal surgeon performing this procedure to be thorough and meticulous. A surgeon with a strong knowledge base and experience, quality surgical technique, and extensive planning can minimize these complications from occurring.

REFERENCES

1. Schwab JA, Pirsig W. Complications of septal surgery. Facial Plast Surg 1997; 13(1):3–14.
2. Muhammad IA, Rahman Nabil-ur. Complications of the surgery for deviated nasal septum. J Coll Physicians Surg Pak 2003;13(10):565–8.
3. Honrado CP, Pastorek NJ. Preventing complications in facial plastic surgery. Curr Opin Otolaryngol Head Neck Surg 2006;14(4):265–9.
4. Bateman ND, Woolford TJ. Informed consent for septal surgery: the evidence-base. J Laryngol Otol 2003;117(3):186–9.
5. Vuyk HD, Langenhuijsen KJ. Aesthetic sequelae of septoplasty. Clin Otolaryngol Allied Sci 1997;22(3):226–32.
6. Slavin SA, Goldwyn RM. The cocaine user: the potential problem patient for rhinoplasty. Plast Reconstr Surg 1990;86(3):436–42.
7. Fedok FG, Ferraro RE, Kingsley CP, et al. Operative times, postanesthesia recovery times, and complications during sinonasal surgery using general anesthesia and local anesthesia with sedation. Otolaryngol Head Neck Surg 2000; 122(4):560–6.
8. Ashchi M, Wiedemann HP, James KB. Cardiac complication from use of cocaine and phenylephrine in nasal septoplasty. Arch Otolaryngol Head Neck Surg 1995; 121(6):681–4.
9. Rettinger G, Kirsche H. Complications in septoplasty. Facial Plast Surg 2006; 22(4):289–97.
10. Ganesan S, Prior AJ, Rubin JS. Unexpected overnight admissions following day-case surgery: an analysis of a dedicated ENT day care unit. Ann R Coll Surg Engl 2000;82(5):327–30.

11. Vaiman M, Sarfaty S, Shlamkovich N, et al. Fibrin sealant: alternative to nasal packing in endonasal operations. A prospective randomized study. Isr Med Assoc J 2005;7(9):571–4 [see comment].
12. Vaiman M, Eviatar E, Segal S. The use of fibrin glue as hemostatic in endonasal operations: a prospective, randomized study. Rhinology 2002;40(4):185–8.
13. Gulsen S, Yilmaz C, Aydin E, et al. Meningoencephalocele formation after nasal septoplasty and management of this complication. Turk Neurosurg 2008;18(3): 281–5.
14. Onerci TM, Ayhan K, Ogretmenoglu O. Two consecutive cases of cerebrospinal fluid rhinorrhea after septoplasty operation. Am J Otolaryngol 2004;25(5):354–6.
15. Tawadros AM, Prahlow JA. Death related to nasal surgery: case report with review of therapy-related deaths. Am J Forensic Med Pathol 2008;29(3):260–4.
16. Makitie A, Aaltonen LM, Hytonen M, et al. Postoperative infection following nasal septoplasty. Acta Otolaryngol Suppl 2000;543:165–6.
17. Okur E, Yildirim I, Aral M, et al. Bacteremia during open septorhinoplasty. Am J Rhinol 2006;20(1):36–9.
18. Caniello M, Passerotti GH, Goto EY, et al. Antibiotics in septoplasty: is it necessary? Rev Bras Otorrinolaringol 2005;71(6):734–8.
19. Uslu H, Uslu C, Varoglu E, et al. Effects of septoplasty and septal deviation on nasal mucociliary clearance. Int J Clin Pract 2004;58(12):1108–11.
20. Eviatar E, Kessler A, Segal S, et al. Effects of septoplasty on the nasal flora. Am J Rhinol 2006;20(1):40–2.
21. Allen ST, Liland JB, Nichols CG, et al. Toxic shock syndrome associated with use of latex nasal packing. Arch Intern Med 1990;150(12):2587–8.
22. Huang IT, Podkomorska D, Murphy MN, et al. Toxic shock syndrome following septoplasty and partial turbinectomy. J Otolaryngol 1986;15(5):310–2.
23. Cohen BJ, Johnson JD, Raff MJ. Septoplasty complicated by staphylococcal spinal osteomyelitis. Arch Intern Med 1985;145(3):556–7.
24. Hari C, Marnane C, Wormald PJ. Quilting sutures for nasal septum. J Laryngol Otol 2008;122(5):522–3.
25. Lee IN, Vukovic L. Hemostatic suture for septoplasty: how we do it. J Otolaryngol 1988;17(1):54–6.
26. Ammar SM, Westreich RW, Lawson W. Fan Septoplasty for Correction of the Internally and Externally Deviated Nose. Arch Facial Plast Surg 2006;8(3):213–6.
27. Byrd SH, Salomon J, Flood J. Correction of the crooked nose. Plast Reconstr Surg 1998;102(6):2148–57.
28. Lee BJ, Chung YS, Jang YJ. Overcorrected septum as a complication of septoplasty. Am J Rhinol 2004;18(6):393–6.
29. Daudia A, Alkhaddour U, Sithole J, et al. A prospective objective study of the cosmetic sequelae of nasal septal surgery. Acta Otolaryngol 2006;126(11): 1201–5.
30. Morre TD, Van Camp C, Clement PA. Results of the endonasal surgical closure of nasoseptal perforations. Acta Otorhinolaryngol Belg 1995;49(3):263–7.
31. Kim DW, Egan KK, O'Grady K, et al. Biomechanical strength of human nasal septal lining: comparison of the constituent layers. Laryngoscope 2005;115(8): 1451–3.
32. Newton JR, White PS, Lee MS. Nasal septal perforation repair using open septoplasty and unilateral bipedicled flaps. J Laryngol Otol 2003;117(1):52–5.
33. Kridel RWH, Foda H, Lunde KC. Septal perforation repair with acellular human dermal allograft. Arch Otolaryngol Head Neck Surg 1998;124:73–8.

34. Ambro BT, Zimmerman J, Rosenthal M, Pribitkin E. Nasal Septal Perforation Repair With Porcine Small Intestinal Submucosa. Arch Facial Plast Surg, Nov 2003;5:528–9.
35. Malki D, Quine SM, Pfleiderer AG. Nasal splints, revisited. J Laryngol Otol 1999; 113(8):725–7.
36. Guyuron B, Vaughan C. Evaluation of stents following septoplasty. Aesthetic Plast Surg 1995;19(1):75–7.
37. Cook JA, Murrant NJ, Evans KL, et al. Intranasal splints and their effects on intranasal adhesions and septal stability. Clin Otolaryngol Allied Sci 1992;17(1):24–7.
38. Hajiioannou JK, Bizaki A, Fragiadakis G, et al. Optimal time for nasal packing removal after septoplasty. A comparative study. Rhinology 2007;45(1):68–71.
39. Yildirim A, Yasar M, Bebek AI, et al. Nasal septal suture technique versus nasal packing after septoplasty. Am J Rhinol 2005;19(6):599–602.
40. Al-Raggad DK, El-Jundi AM, Al-Momani OS, et al. Suturing of the nasal septum after septoplasty, is it an effective alternative to nasal packing? Saudi Med J 2007;28(10):1534–6.
41. Briner HR, Simmen D, Jones N. Impaired sense of smell in patients with nasal surgery. Clin Otolaryngol Allied Sci 2003;28(5):417–9.
42. Chandra RK, Rohman GT, Walsh WE. Anterior palate sensory impairment after septal surgery. Am J Rhinol 2008;22(1):86–8.
43. Guyuron B, Michelow B, Thomas T. Gustatory rhinorrhea—a complication of septoplasty. Plast Reconstr Surg 1994;94(3):454–6.
44. Monteiro ML. Unilateral blindness as a complication of nasal septoplasty: case report. Arq Bras Oftalmol 2006;69(2):249–50.

Surgical Management of the Septal Perforation

Deborah Watson, MD, FACS*, Gregory Barkdull, MD

KEYWORDS

- Septal perforation repair • Septal repair flaps
- Septal perforation management • Septal injury
- Septal inflammation • Septal button

Nasal septal perforations are relatively common, affecting up to 0.9% of the general population.[1] The challenge for the rhinologic or nasal reconstructive surgeon is to identify those cases that require additional work-up and to select the medical and surgical treatments most appropriate for the patient at hand.

Most symptomatic perforations are located at the anterior septum, which is composed of three layers: the anterior part of the quadrangular cartilage and the bilateral layers of mucoperichondrium. Although the blood supply to this region is redundant and includes branches from both the external carotid and internal carotid arteries, vasculitis or trauma to the terminal branches of the septum can devitalize the nasal septal mucosa. When the mucoperichondrium becomes ischemic, the underlying cartilaginous septum quickly necroses. After a perforation has formed, the mucosal edges quickly epithelialize, and this process prevents closure of the defect during normal healing.[2]

In the presence of a perforation, the normal intranasal laminar airflow becomes altered, producing symptoms that include whistling, crusting, and nasal airway obstruction. Furthermore, the persistence of dry nasal crust, coupled with chronic manipulation of it, can lead to progressive enlargement of the defect.

Complications can arise from undiagnosed, severe, or inadequately treated cases of septal perforation. Low-grade perichondritis can occur in cases associated with poor hygiene. Epistaxis can result from a patient picking at or removing crusted, dried mucous secretions that collect at the edges of the perforation, or from granulation tissue at this site. Finally, the progression of an enlarging anterior septal perforation will eventually cause deterioration of the dorsal and caudal septal support of the

Division of Otolaryngology-Head and Neck Surgery, UCSD School of Medicine, 3350 La Jolla Village Dr., 112-C, San Diego, CA 92161, USA
* Corresponding author.
E-mail address: debwatson@ucsd.edu (D. Watson).

Otolaryngol Clin N Am 42 (2009) 483–493
doi:10.1016/j.otc.2009.03.011
0030-6665/09/$ – see front matter. Published by Elsevier Inc.

nose. The impact of this effect is not only a functional problem of nasal airway obstruction from vestibular stenosis or internal nasal valve collapse, but it is also an aesthetic issue of nasal tip collapse and/or saddle-nose deformity.

EVALUATION

Although most septal perforations are iatrogenic, traumatic or drug-induced, there are a few cases that are caused by inflammatory conditions, malignancy, and infectious disease (**Box 1**). It is prudent to determine the underlying etiology before recommending a surgical repair.

This process begins with a careful history. The chief complaint may include nasal airway obstruction, an audible whistle during nasal breathing, nasal crusting, intranasal pain, epistaxis, or foul and copious nasal discharge. Advanced cases may present with a saddle-nose deformity. The onset of the perforation and attributing circumstances should be explored. Pertinent details include any prior nasal procedures including cautery, septoplasty, and cosmetic surgery. The inquiry should include events of prior trauma, cocaine use, excessive use of vasoconstrictors, or intranasal injury from foreign bodies. A complete evaluation should inquire about risk factors for tuberculosis and syphilis, as well as occupational exposures, including chemical irritants and particulates. The patient should be queried about their nasal hygiene habits; whether they perform sinonasal irrigation, apply ointment intranasally, use intranasal sprays, or digitally remove nasal crusts.

After a complete head and neck examination, nasal endoscopy is recommended to provide the surgeon with improved visualization of the anatomic details. The edges of the perforation can be assessed for active ulceration (associated with raw granulation or fibrinous tissue) or evidence of healing with well-epithelialized edges. The size of the perforation should be determined as this can influence the selection of repair technique for some surgeons. Measurements of the perforation can be performed in several ways. The diameter of the endoscopic lens can be used as a measuring tool from one edge of the perforation to the other. The end of a centimeter-etched Cottle elevator can be carefully inserted and slid against the septum to determine the size of the perforation. The disposable paper ruler found in some surgical pen packs can be trimmed and introduced into the nose to obtain an accurate measurement. Finally, a trained eye can provide a close estimate of the defect. If the perforation is not uniformly circular, it is helpful to measure the vertical height of a perforation as well as the anterior–posterior dimension, because this may also affect the choice of surgical repair. The final feature to take note of is the location of the perforation: anterior, posterior, low near the floor or high near dorsum.

Further laboratory evaluation can be useful after the history and physical examination help to narrow the differential diagnosis. Churg-Strauss syndrome is identified by an elevated perinuclear-staining antineutrophil cytoplasmic antibodies (p-ANCA) and peripheral blood eosinophilia. Patients with Wegener's granulomatosis often have elevated antineutrophil cytoplasmic autoantibody (c-ANCA) levels, as well as elevated erythrocyte sedimentation rate (ESR) and rheumatoid factor (RF), but these latter tests are less specific.[3] The serum angiotensin-converting enzyme (ACE) level is elevated along with serum calcium levels in patients with sarcoid. They may also exhibit mediastinal adenopathy on chest radiograph. In patients who have active and inflamed lesions of the septum, the posterior edge of the perforation should be biopsied; the tissue can be sent for pathology as well as acid-fast bacilli and fungal cultures. Biopsies of the superior margin of the perforation should be avoided because they contribute to the vertical diameter of the defect and increase the difficulty of the

| **Box 1** |
| **Differential diagnosis for septal perforation** |

Iatrogenic

    Septoplasty

    Rhinoplasty

    Nasal cautery

    Nasal intubation

Traumatic

    Mucosal laceration

    Digital trauma

    Septal hematoma

    Foreign body

Inflammatory

    Sarcoidosis

    Churg-Strauss syndrome

    Wegener's granulomatosis

    Lupus

Infectious

    Invasive fungal infection

    Septal abscess

    Tuberculosis

    Syphilis

Malignancy

    Lymphoma

Inhalants

    Intranasal steroids

    Cocaine

    Sulfuric acid fumes

    Glass dust

    Mercurials

    Phosphorus

    Vasoconstrictive nasal sprays

eventual closure. Finally, a sinus CT scan can be helpful to look for co-existing sinus disease and serve as an aid in preoperative sizing of the perforation.

NONSURGICAL TREATMENT
Nasal Hygiene

Initial management of septal perforation begins with improving nasal hygiene and counseling the patient to avoid digital cleaning. Routine nasal irrigation with saline solution or regular humidification can help reduce the build-up of crusts. Antibiotic ointment or any petroleum-based ointment can prevent the drying and hardening of crusted material, as long as the ointment is applied intranasally a few times daily. In the setting of visible mucosal inflammation, an antibiotic-based ointment might be preferable. Patients who have complaints of pain and dryness at the perforation site often experience improved comfort when the ointment is used to lubricate and soothe the mucous membranes within the nasal vestibule and anterior septum. Despite these measures, some of the symptomatic complaints of the patient may remain unresolved, and the risk of progressive enlargement of the perforation is always present.

Nasal Septal Button

Temporary closure of the perforation can be achieved with a nasal septal button. This prosthetic device can be inserted into position during an office visit with the aid of local or topical anesthesia and decongestant. To facilitate proper placement, one side of the disk is folded and passed or pulled through the perforation with alligator or bayonet forceps. An endoscopic view of the nasal cavity may facilitate this maneuver. The flanges should fit into the region of the internal nasal valve superiorly and come in contact with the nasal floor inferiorly. These buttons are commercially available in various sizes. After a septal button is inserted, it can remain in place for one year or more, but this duration is very dependent on the patient's diligence with good nasal hygiene and proper care of the prosthesis. Indications for device removal include: the need to size-up the prosthesis; the relief of chronic discomfort from the button; and to enable ongoing cleaning and maintenance.

Unfortunately, septal buttons have been associated with several complications. In some patients, they increase the frequency of epistaxis, can allow crusted material to collect around the flanges, cause intranasal pain, and may contribute to a steady erosion of the perforation edges and eventual enlargement of the defect.

SURGICAL TREATMENT

First and foremost the surgeon and patient should remember that septal perforation repair is elective. With appropriate and conservative methods of intranasal irrigation and ointment application, a patient can minimize some of their symptoms, and may slow or prevent further enlargement of the perforation. However, there is always the potential for the defect to worsen with time, and create additional problems for the patient. Because small perforations have higher rates of successful surgical closure than larger perforations, there is a theoretical advantage to early repair.[4]

The goals of a surgical repair are to: provide as much of a tension-free closure as possible, restore normal nasal function, and in some cases, reconstruct nasal support. The success of surgery depends on several variables: the height and location of the perforation, the amount of remaining cartilage, the presence of mucosal scar tissue, and the experience and skill of the surgeon.

Presurgical Considerations

Current use of cocaine is an absolute contraindication to surgery because the repair will invariably fail. In one author's experience, only 10% of cocaine users were able to stop the use of cocaine and, thus, the author recommends a psychiatric evaluation before offering surgery.[5] It may also be necessary to confirm with preoperative blood testing that patients have indeed stopped their cocaine use. Not only are these patients prone to surgical site failure, they are also at increased risk for anesthetic complications.[4] Surgery should be delayed until patients have demonstrated that they are no longer using and all raw ulcerations have healed. There is no consensus on the appropriate timing of repair for patients with Wegener's granulomatosis, but the general wisdom is to defer surgery until the patient is in remission and the active ulcerations have healed.

Endonasal Approach

Small defects less than 5 mm can be closed by the endonasal approach. These repairs typically begin with a hemitransfixion incision, followed by adequate elevation of the mucoperichondrial flaps dorsally, ventrally and finally posteriorly. Before the reapproximation of the septal mucosal flaps with basting sutures, an interpositional graft can be inserted to reinforce the repair. Choices for interpositional graft material include bone, cartilage, periosteum and acellular dermal allograft (Alloderm, Life-Cell Corp., Branchburg, New Jersey). Alloderm, in particular, has gained popularity as an interpositional graft in septal perforation repair due to its availability and ease of use.[6] It is cut to a size larger than the perforation and then inserted between the mucoperichondrial flaps. Generous elevation of the mucoperichondrium will provide enough laxity of the membrane to permit apposition or overlap of the perforation edges. During the placement of basting sutures, care should be taken to conceal the interpositional graft. By staggering the closure, one can avoid overlapping suture lines. Postoperative care is similar to other techniques, with the use of silastic splints for 2 to 3 weeks followed by careful nasal hygiene.

External Rhinoplasty Approach

Although some authors have successfully closed moderately-sized perforations (5 mm to 2 cm) with an endonasal approach,[7–9] the open rhinoplasty approach provides superior access, greater mucoperichondrial mobilization and an overall higher success rate of 90% or greater.[2,4] This approach is described in detail in the following paragraphs.

First, the nose is decongested and local anesthetic infiltrated along the septum and into the skin-soft-tissue envelope (SSTE) of the middle and lower nasal vaults, as is typical for an open rhinoplasty approach. After an inverted-v midcolumellar and bilateral marginal incisions are made, dissection proceeds in the subperichondrial plane to elevate the SSTE from the lower and upper lateral cartilages. At this point, the lower lateral cartilages are retracted laterally to permit further dissection toward the anterior septal angle. The interdomal ligament and soft tissue attachments of the medial crura are divided as the septal mucosal flaps are developed.

Dissection

Meticulous dissection is essential as the region of the perforation is reached. Each flap that is developed will be thin, and the potential to enlarge the perforation further is high. Elevation of the mucoperichondrium should extend posteriorly to expose the bony septum, and inferiorly to expose the maxillary crest and nasal floor to the junction of the hard and soft palate. There are often dense fibers near the maxillary crest that have to be incised sharply to avoid laceration of the flap. The floor dissection should extend laterally to the insertion of the inferior turbinate bone to the lateral nasal wall. Any deviated septal cartilage or bone is straightened or removed, as this will provide greater laxity of the membrane by eliminating areas that "tent up" the mucous membrane. Next, a lateral releasing incision is made, just below the insertion of the inferior turbinate to the lateral nasal sidewall. The extent of the lateral incision can span the length of the inferior turbinate (**Fig. 1**). A bipedicled flap is effectively created, which a bipedicled mucoperichondrial flap, which can be medially advanced to close the perforation (**Fig. 2**). If mucosal mobility is limited, or the defect cannot be closed

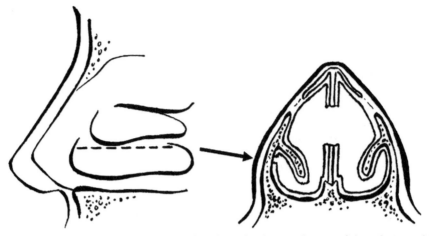

Fig. 1. Lateral releasing incision is placed directly under the attachment of the inferior turbinate bone to the lateral nasal wall.

with this maneuver alone, then a transverse mucosal incision is necessary to provide additional mucosal release. This incision extends from the nasal spine, runs across the anterior nasal sill, and is directed toward the lateral wall of the pyriform aperture. At the level of the inferior turbinate insertion, the transverse incision connects with the lateral incision in a right angle fashion (**Fig. 3**). The bipedicled flap becomes converted to a rotational flap design with this last maneuver. When the defect is larger, and difficult to close with the above-mentioned incisions, additional mucosal mobility is possible by carefully separating the mucoperichondrium from the undersurface of the lower lateral cartilages, and recruiting the mucoperichondrium from areas above the septal defect. This permits recruitment of the mucoperichondrium from areas above the defect (**Fig. 4**).

Defect closure
Depending on the direction of mucosal laxity and flap movement, closure of the defect is verified by gently pulling the edges together using fine toothed-forceps. Before

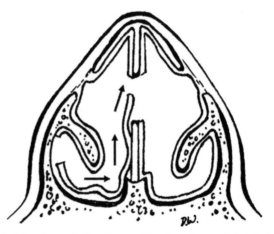

Fig. 2. The bipedicled flap is medially advanced to close the septal defect.

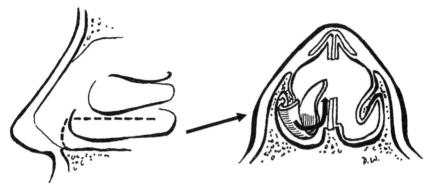

Fig. 3. Transverse releasing incision is placed along the nasal sill; it joins the anterior extent of the lateral releasing incision.

suture repair, a piece of foil from a suture or scalpel package is cut into a circular shape, slightly larger than the defect. The foil barrier is inserted in between the two layers of mucoperichondrium, to prevent the tip of the needle from snagging the contralateral flap during the suturing process. The defect on each mucosal side is closed separately with 5–0 chromic in a running or interrupted fashion, from posterior to anterior. A tapered needle can be helpful in minimizing the tendency of the mucosa to tear when a cutting needle is used.

Graft placement
Before the interpositional graft is placed, the foil barrier is removed. If Alloderm is the preferred graft material, a medium or thick sheet is adequate, but the size of the sheet must exceed the size of the defect. The acellular dermal graft can be trimmed either in its dehydrated state or after the two saline baths that are recommended by the manufacturer. Placement of the graft is facilitated by forceps or a Cottle elevator. Care must be taken to ensure that the graft lays flat and generously spans the area of mucosal repair. A 4–0 plain gut on a straight needle is used to reapproximate the mucosal flaps.

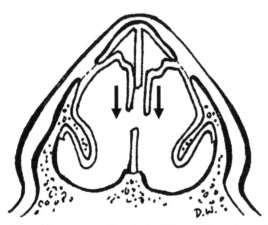

Fig. 4. The mucoperichondrium can be dissected off the undersurface of the upper lateral cartilages, to facilitate closure of the defect by additional mucosal recruitment from above.

As the mucoperichondrium is carefully basted together, several passes of the suture through the graft location will help to secure it in position.

Repositioning

In most cases, the lower lateral cartilages require simple re-approximation with horizontal mattress sutures in between the medial crura and interdomal sutures. Accommodations might need to be made for placement of a columellar strut in situations involving tip ptosis. When significant mucosal recruitment is necessary, it will have a secondary effect of rotating the intermediate crus when the perforation is closed. For many patients, this result would be an undesired aesthetic outcome; therefore, the domal position of the lower lateral cartilages is reset with carefully placed intradomal horizontal mattress sutures. Suitable sutures for cartilage re-positioning can include 5–0 PDS-II (Ethicon, Somerville, New Jersey) or 5–0 Maxon (Covidien, Mansfield, Massachusetts).

Incision closure

After the SSTE is replaced back into position, the closure of the columellar and marginal incisions proceed in the usual manner for an open rhinoplasty approach. The areas of exposed nasal floor that result from rotation of the mucous membrane are left to re-mucosalize. This result occurs successfully with appropriate postoperative care. Bilateral silastic intranasal splints (Doyle Splints, Medtronic, Minneapolis, Minnesota) are lubricated with antibiotic ointment, and placed carefully against the septum. The silastic splints are secured in the region of the anterior septum with a 2–0 monofilament suture. An external nasal cast can be applied at the conclusion of the surgery and left in place for 5 to 7 days. The intranasal Doyle splints are typically removed between 2 to 3 weeks postoperatively, and the patients are instructed to avoid nose blowing for the first month. Gentle saline irrigation with frequent intranasal application of a petroleum-based ointment will facilitate softening and loosening of nasal crusts. This hydrating intranasal environment will also encourage re-mucosalization of the nasal floor. Additional follow-up is suggested to monitor the patient's healing progress several weeks later.

Closure of larger perforations

Perforations larger than 2 cm are more difficult to close with local, intranasal flaps. An array of alternative flaps has been described in the literature. Options include the inferior turbinate pedicled flap, the tunneled sublabial mucosal flap, the facial artery musculomucosal flap (FAMM), and the radial forearm-facial free flap. A brief description of these flaps is included below. A final option for large septal perforations is to perform a staged tissue expansion followed by reconstruction of the defect 2 weeks later, using either an external rhinoplasty or midfacial degloving approach.[10]

Inferior Turbinate Pedicled Flap

The inferior turbinate flap has utility in repairing perforations of the caudal septum up to 2.0 cm in diameter[11] and can be performed through an endonasal approach. An advantage of this flap is that it can reach a defect that involves the columella. A through-and-through incision is made at the posterior–inferior aspect of the turbinate. The flap includes mucosa and submucosa, and it can incorporate a variable amount of bone if needed. The distal portion of the flap is pulled forward and split open. It is then sutured into the septal perforation with 4–0 or 5–0 plain gut suture. Because the ipsilateral side has the advantage of the mucosal covering, the contralateral septal surface bears the exposed raw submucosa that will heal by secondary intention. This flap procedure requires a second stage to divide the pedicle. The division is performed 3 weeks later, in an outpatient setting under local anesthetic. Contraindications to this technique include prior turbinate surgery and atrophic rhinitis. Reported complications of this technique include nasal obstruction from the bulk of the flap, adhesions between the septum and the remaining inferior turbinate, and a small possibility of complete flap necrosis.[5]

Tunneled Sublabial Mucosal Flap

The sublabial mucosal flap has been advocated by Tardy for closure of large anterior perforations.[12] This procedure uses the relatively abundant oral mucosa by making an incision in the ipsilateral buccal mucosa. A medially-based pedicled flap is raised that is 20% larger than the defect. The mucosal is left intact adjacent to the frenulum. A midline sublabial-nasal fistula is created with sharp dissection and the flap is brought up into the nose and tunneled between the previously elevated septal mucoperichondrial flaps. A disadvantage to this flap is that it can result in a persistent oral nasal fistula and if there is pressure on the tunneled mucosa, the flap can necrose.

Facial Artery Musculomucosal Flap

One regional pedicled flap that has been used with success is the facial artery musculomucosal (FAMM) flap.[13] This flap can be used to close perforations 2 to 4 cm in size. The flap is based on retrograde flow through the facial artery. The donor area is the buccal mucosa immediately subjacent to the facial artery and extends to the inferior gingivobuccal sulcus. Using an intraoperative Doppler can aid in designing the flap. It is then harvested along with the underlying vessel and then tunneled through a subperiosteal dissection into the piriform aperture where it is sewn into position. The contralateral side of the peforation can be skin grafted or let to granulate. Because the buccal mucosa is freely transferred, there is less chance of fistula formation than with the tunneled sublabial flap. One of the limitations that the authors report is that patients can have some cheek tightness in the donor site, but it usually resolves with time and massage.[14]

Radial Forearm Free Flap

The radial forearm free flap is based on the radial artery, which can be anastamosed to the facial artery and sewn into the nasal septal defect. Several authors have reported success closing large defects.[15,16] Although this flap provides plenty of vascularized dermis for the reconstruction, obvious drawbacks include the inherent difficulties of microvascular anastomosis, length of time involved in performing the procedure, significant donor site morbidity, and the problems associated with nasal dryness secondary to the dermal lining within the nose.

AESTHETIC CONSIDERATIONS

Larger septal perforations or those close to the columella may contribute to saddle-nose deformity or tip collapse. Fortunately, nasal structure defects can be corrected at the time that the perforation is repaired. Anecdotally, nasal reconstructive surgeons have preferred the use of autologous cartilage to rebuild the nasal structure. In a few cases, there may be adequate septal cartilage remaining that can be harvested for structural grafting. Auricular cartilage grafts are an option; however, auricular cartilage does not offer the length, contour or stiffness that is needed in many nasal reconstructive cases. Reconstructive nasal surgeons may gravitate to harvesting costal cartilage because there is adequate supply of this tissue source. Rib cartilage provides the length, stiffness, and proper contours for cartilage grafting after it is appropriately

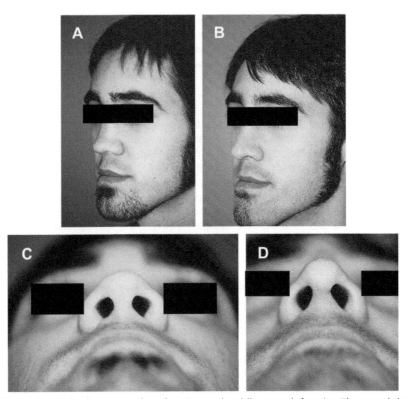

Fig. 5. A patient who has a septal perforation and saddle-nose deformity. The septal defect was repaired using an external rhinoplasty approach, bilateral mucosal flaps, and an interpositional graft. The dorsal deformity and poor tip support were corrected with autologous rib cartilage. A dorsal graft and a columella strut were inserted and stabilized with sutures. (*A*) Preoperative oblique view; (*B*) postoperative oblique view; (*C*) preoperative base view; (*D*) postoperative base view.

sculpted into the required graft shape and size (**Fig. 5**). Autologous cartilage has an advantage over synthetic implants in that it does not contribute to graft rejection or extrusion. Using autologous rib cartilage does require experience and skill in sculpting, and unfortunately, this cartilage type carries a low risk of warping.

The technical steps for costal cartilage harvesting and saddle-nose deformity repair is beyond the scope of this article. However, when planning out the grafts, their stabilization within the nasal framework is critical. The cartilage grafts are placed into precise soft tissue pockets, suturing them to existing nasal cartilage, or interlocking them to one another.

SUMMARY

Successful management of septal perforation begins with a careful history and examination. After the etiology has been determined and the predisposing condition dealt with, a treatment plan can be developed for the patient. Options for surgical closure of the perforation are related to the size and location of the perforation. The majority of small, anterior septal perforations less than 0.5 cm can be successfully closed endonasally. Larger defects benefit from the open rhinoplasty approach. Although there are several flap choices that can be used with the latter approach, the selection of bilateral mucosal advancement with an interpositional graft tends to have the greatest success.

REFERENCES

1. Oberg D, Akerlund A, Johansson L, et al. Prevalence of nasal septal perforation: the Skövde population-based study. Rhinology 2003;41(2):72–5.
2. Kridel RW. Septal perforation repair. Rhinoplasty and septoplasty, part II. Otolaryngol Clin North Am 1999;32(4):695–724.
3. Diamantopoulos II, Jones NS. The investigation of nasal septal perforations and ulcers. J Laryngol Otol 2001;115(7):541–4.
4. Kridel RW. Considerations in the etiology, treatment, and repair of septal perforations. Facial Plast Surg Clin North Am 2004;12:435–50.
5. Pedroza F, Patrocinio LG, Arevalo O. A review of 25-year experience of nasal septal perforation repair. Arch Facial Plast Surg 2007;9:12–8.
6. Kridel RW, Foda H, Lunde KC. Septal perforation repair with acellular human dermal allograft. Arch Otolaryngol Head Neck Surg 1998;124(1):73–8.
7. Tasca I, Compadretti GC. Closure of nasal septal perforation via endonasal approach. Otolaryngol Head Neck Surg 2006;135(6):922–7.
8. Fairbanks DN. Closure of nasal septal perforations. Arch Otolaryngol 1980; 106(8):509–13.
9. Fairbanks DN, Fairbanks GR. Nasal septal perforation: prevention and management. Ann Plast Surg 1980;5(6):452–9.
10. Romo T, Yalamanchili H, Presti P, et al. Septal perforation: surgical aspects. eMedicine 2007.
11. Friedman M, Ibrahim H, Ramakrishnan V. Inferior turbinate flap for repair of nasal septal perforation. Laryngoscope 2003;113(8):1425–8.
12. Tardy ME. Practical suggestions on facial plastic surgery–how I do it. Sublabial mucosal flap: repair of septal perforations. Laryngoscope 1977;87(2):275–8.
13. Pribaz J, Stephens W, Crespo L, et al. New intraoral flap: facial artery musculomucosal (FAMM) flap. Plast Reconstr Surg 1992;90(3):421–9.
14. Heller JB, Gabbay JS, Trussler A. Repair of large septal perforations using facial artery musculomucosal (FAMM) flap. Ann Plast Surg 2005;55:456–9.
15. Mobley SR, Boyd JB, Astor FC. Repair of a large septal perforation with a radial forearm free flap: brief report of a case. Ear Nose Throat J 2001;80(8):512.
16. Barry C, Eadie PA, Russell J. Radial forearm free flap for repair of a large nasal septal perforation: a report of a case in a child. J Plast Reconstr Aesthet Surg 2008;61(8):996–7.

Surgical and Nonsurgical Treatments of the Nasal Valves

Judy Lee, MD, W. Matthew White, MD, Minas Constantinides, MD, FACS*

KEYWORDS

- Functional rhinoplasty • Internal nasal valve
- External nasal valve • Nasal obstruction • Spreader grafts
- Batten grafts • Alar strut grafts

Nasal obstruction is known to be associated with a major decrease in disease-specific quality of life, and nasal valve dysfunction can play a considerable role in nasal airflow obstruction.[1] Diagnosis and treatment of nasal valve dysfunction requires a thorough understanding of normal anatomy and function and pathophysiology of common abnormalities to properly treat the exact source of dysfunction.

ANATOMY

First described by Mink[2] in 1903, the term "nasal valve" has been used to describe the main site of nasal resistance, which he initially described as a "slit-like opening" placed at the junction between the upper lateral cartilages (ULC) and the lower lateral cartilages (LLC). Historically, the internal valve has been defined as the area between the caudal end of the ULC and the cartilaginous septum. This angle is typically 10 to 15 degrees in the Caucasian nose, and more obtuse in the African American or Asian nose. A more contemporary, three-dimensional description includes the ULC superiorly, cartilaginous septum medially, head of the inferior turbinate posteriorly, nasal floor inferiorly, and nasal alar and bony pyriform aperture laterally in the nasal valve area.[3] Today, the nasal valve is further divided into an internal and external component. The external nasal valve is described as the cross-sectional area caudal to the internal valve under the alar lobule, bounded superolaterally by the caudal edge of the ULC, laterally by the nasal alar and ligamentous attachment of the lateral crus, medially by the caudal septum and columella, and inferiorly by the nasal sill. The

Division of Facial Plastic and Reconstructive Surgery, Department of Otolaryngology, Head and Neck Surgery, New York University School of Medicine, 530 First Avenue, Suite 7U, New York, NY 10016, USA
* Corresponding author.
E-mail address: minas.constantinides@med.nyu.edu (M. Constantinides).

Otolaryngol Clin N Am 42 (2009) 495–511
doi:10.1016/j.otc.2009.03.010
0030-6665/09/$ – see front matter © 2009 Elsevier Inc. All rights reserved.

primary muscles responsible for maintaining the patency of the external nasal valve include the nasalis and dilator naris muscles.

A contemporary classification system of the internal nasal valve has been described by Miman and colleagues,[4] using endoscopic evaluation to describe various valve characteristics, including convex, concave, sharp angle, blunt angle, twisted caudal border, and angle occupied by the septal body. They found that the internal nasal-valve angle occupied by the septal body was found to have increased nasal resistances compared with the sharp-angled internal nasal-valve type. The authors designated classification groups according to either the upper cartilage's caudal border status (convex, concave, or twisted), or the angle status (blunt, sharp, or occupied by the septal body).

PHYSIOLOGY

The cross-sectional area of the nasal valve is between 55 to 83 mm^2 and is the main site of greatest nasal resistance. It functions as the primary regulator of airflow and resistance, providing the sensation of normal airway patency. As described by Poiseuille's law, nasal resistance is inversely proportional to the radius of the nasal passages raised to the fourth power (resistance = [viscosity * length]/$radius^4$). Small changes in the cross-sectional area of the nasal valve produce exponential effects on airflow and resistance.

The nasal valve functions as a Starling resistor, which consists of a semirigid tube with a collapsible segment anteriorly, and collapses with forceful inspiration to limit airflow. As described by the Bernoulli principle, the degree of lateral sidewall collapse depends on the intrinsic stability of the valve and on the transmural pressure changes during normal and forceful inspiration. As flow increases through a fixed space or volume, pressure in that fixed space decreases. As airflow velocity increases, the pressure inside the nasal valve decreases relative to atmospheric pressure, thus increasing the transmural pressure difference. As this transmural difference increases, the likelihood of nasal valve collapse increases. This may be a protective mechanism to prevent large volumes of unheated and unhumidified air from reaching the lower respiratory tract. In individuals with either acquired or congenital valve collapse, this mechanism functions at a transmural pressure that is too low and can lead to premature collapse and difficulty with nasal breathing. Partial collapse of the ULC normally occurs at a respiratory flow rate of 30 L/min, preventing further increases in intranasal pressure from increasing flow.

Nasal valve obstruction can be further divided into static and dynamic dysfunction. Static dysfunction is caused by continuous obstruction at the level of the nasal valve because of structural and skeletal deformities, such as inferior turbinate hypertrophy, deviated nasal septum, cicatricle stenosis, or medially displaced ULC. Static dysfunction requires more intranasal pressure to generate a given amount of nasal airflow. Dynamic dysfunction, in contrast, is caused by collapsible or deficient structural support of the nasal sidewall, including the cartilaginous, fibrofatty, and muscular components, resulting in collapse of the nasal valve at low transmural pressures.

ETIOLOGIES

As described by Kern and Wang,[5] the etiologies of nasal valve dysfunction can be classified as mucocutaneous or structural/skeletal abnormalities. Conditions that can cause mucosal inflammation and edema, contributing to nasal valve obstruction, include sinusitis, nasal polyposis, and all forms of rhinitis ranging from allergic to vasomotor to infectious. Structural or skeletal causes of nasal valve obstruction include any deformities of individual components of the nasal valve complex. These may include the nasal septum, upper and lower lateral cartilages, fibrofatty sidewall tissue, pyriform aperture, and floor of nose.

Static structural deformities of the internal nasal valve can be caused by inferomedially displaced ULC, narrowed pyriform aperture, scarring at the intercartilaginous junction, deviated nasal septum, and inferior turbinate hypertrophy. Dynamic deformities are often secondary to destabilization of the septum and LLC, resulting in ULC collapse. Static abnormalities of the external nasal valve can be caused by tip ptosis, cicatricle stenosis, or caudal septal deviations, whereas dynamic deformities include musculature deficiencies and either primary or postoperative LLC weaknesses.

Previous nasal surgeries, namely reduction rhinoplasties, can contribute significantly to nasal valve obstruction. Grymer[6] showed that the cross-sectional area at the nasal valve decreased by 25% and the pyriform aperture by 11% to 13% using acoustic rhinometry after reduction rhinoplasty. A recent retrospective review of 53 subjects by Khosh and colleagues[7] showed that previous rhinoplasty was the cause of nasal valve obstruction in 79% of subjects, followed by nasal trauma (15%) and congenital anomaly (6%).

Several rhinoplasty techniques can contribute to postrhinoplasty nasal valve dysfunction. Overaggressive dorsal hump reductions that destabilize the ULC, and surgical over-resections of the LLC, may lead to collapse of the nasal sidewall. Scroll release with knuckling may also occur with overaggressive cephalic trims of the LLC and caudal trims of the ULC. Bossa formation at the nasal tip can occur with scroll release, tip-graft migration, or excessive postoperative scarring, especially in patients with preexisting bifidity or stiff LLC, all of which can lead to nasal valve obstruction postrhinoplasty.

Sheen described that with resection of the middle vault roof, the flaccid ULC, once disarticulated from the nasal septum, tends to fall inferomedially toward the nasal septum. This results in a narrowed middle vault characteristically described as the inverted-V deformity.[8] This may lead to dynamic and static collapse of the ULC caused by their disarticulation from the septum medially, decreasing nasal valve areas, and more readily allowing dynamic collapse with inspiration. Traumatic displacement of the nasal bones, ULC, LLC, or nasal septum is a leading cause of acquired nasal valve dysfunction. When nasal fractures are being repaired, mobilizing and correcting the nasal bones and the attached cephalic border of the ULCs should be accomplished before correction of the internal nasal valve.[9]

Other causes of nasal valve dysfunction include tip ptosis, cicatricial stenosis, facial paralysis, and paradoxical lateral crura.[9] Tip ptosis can be from excess soft-tissue bulk causing narrowing of the nasal vestibule or structural ptosis secondary to saddle nose deformity or weakened LLC medial crura postrhinoplasty. Cicatricial stenosis is an uncommon cause of external nasal valve obstruction and is usually iatrogenic. Facial paralysis can result in collapse of the nasal sidewall caused by loss of muscular tone of the dilator naris and nasalis muscles. Paradoxical lateral crura describes a rare phenomenon where the LLC lack normal external convexity in the lateral crura. These abnormal cartilages may project into the nasal vestibule causing static obstruction and dynamic obstruction with decreased resistance to collapse during inspiration.

EVALUATION OF THE PATIENT

When evaluating a patient for nasal obstruction, a thorough history and systematic physical examination is taken to determine appropriate management. Once the source of nasal obstruction is determined and is amenable to surgery, there are three areas of the nose that are typically involved that require evaluation: the medial nasal wall, the lateral wall, and the nasal valves. Constantinides, Galli, and Miller describe[10] a simple, systematic method of patient evaluation examining these three areas so that surgical treatment can be modified to address the specific anatomic deformity. Preoperative evaluation includes a detailed intranasal examination with a nasal speculum and nasal endoscopy. The Cottle maneuver has been well described in the evaluation of nasal obstruction, where the cheek and lateral nostril are displaced laterally to assess for improved nasal airflow. A modified Cottle maneuver using a small ear curette that examines two separate areas of nasal support, lower lateral cartilage and upper lateral cartilage, can be performed to assess specific deficiencies.

First, the patient is asked to rate their breathing on a 0- to 10-scale, with 0 indicating complete nasal obstruction, and 10 indicating clear inspiration. Each side is rated independently, with the side that is not being rated gently occluded. Then, the ear curette is used to elevate the LLC and then the ULC, just enough to mimic the support that is expected with surgical grafting. At each level of support, the patient is asked again to rate the breathing on the same 0- to 10-scale. Improved nasal airflow with LLC support suggests that the external nasal valve needs grafting. Improved nasal patency with ULC support suggests a need for internal nasal valve correction. This maneuver should be done before and after decongestant therapy. These examination findings help guide the proper management of nasal valve dysfunction.

NONSURGICAL TREATMENTS OF NASAL VALVE OBSTRUCTION

Nonsurgical and medical interventions for the treatment of nasal valve dysfunction are appropriate for many patients with mild or mucosal etiologies for their dysfunction. Patients with mild-structural dysfunction or those that are poor surgical candidates may find relief with commercial nasal valve dilators, such as Breathe-Right strips (CNS Inc., Minneapolis, Minnesota). A newer nonsurgical technique described by Nyte[11] for correcting nasal valve collapse is a spreader graft like injection with calcium hydroxylapatite (Radiesse, BioForm Medical, Franksville, Wisconsin) into the submucoperichondrial or submucosal plane at points on the ULC and at the junction between the dorsal septum and ULC. This may lateralize the ULC, making it less likely to collapse with inspiration. The author notes successful spreader graft injection in 23 subjects to date, with minimal adverse effects with follow-up ranging from 3 to 10 months, although percentages are not provided. All patients reported subjective improvement in nasal patency or alleviation of snoring.

Patients with symptoms that improve significantly with nasal-decongestant therapy or those associated with inflammatory or infectious processes, should be treated medically, at least initially, but may require surgical intervention for refractory cases. A recent retrospective review by Inanli examining 45 subjects who underwent concurrent functional endoscopic sinus surgery and rhinoplasty demonstrated that combined surgery may be done safely without major complication, may be more cost-effective, and yield pleasing aesthetic and functional outcomes.[12]

SURGICAL TREATMENTS OF NASAL VALVE DYSFUNCTION

If a patient has exhausted medical management and the site of obstruction is identified, a surgical treatment plan specific to the dysfunctional element is determined. Nasal septal deviations and inferior turbinate hypertrophy can significantly contribute to obstruction of the nasal valve complex and should be addressed at the time of surgery, either alone or in conjunction with additional nasal surgery.[9] Many authors will agree that septoplasty for anterior septal deviation is beneficial. Hypertrophic inferior turbinates can be reduced in multiple ways, including submucous resection, KTP laser, coblation, and radiofrequency ablation, with or without outfracturing.

Internal nasal-valve abnormalities can be corrected with a number of surgical techniques. One may choose to perform these maneuvers with an open or endonasal approach, depending on surgeon preference. The mainstay of treatment has included spreader grafts, harvested from septal, or less favorably, conchal cartilage, which are placed in a submucosal pocket between the septum and the ULC.[8] These grafts are typically 1- to 2- mm thick and extend the full length of the ULC. They are fixed in place with horizontal-mattress sutures that span the ULC, spreader graft or grafts, and dorsal septum. Trimming or tapering of the graft may be necessary to remove excess cartilage that may be visible or palpable (**Fig. 1**).

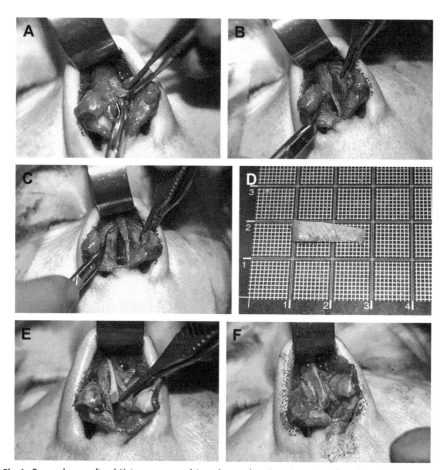

Fig. 1. Spreader grafts. (*A*) In an open rhinoplasty, the tip scissors is placed in the submucoperichondrial pocket between the left ULC and the septum. (*B*) The left ULC has been cut away sharply from the dorsal septum. The forceps is holding the left ULC laterally. (*C*) Both ULC have been sharply cut away from the dorsal septum, leaving the overlying mucoperichondrium intact. (*D*) A typical spreader graft. Note the fine tapering at the end that will insert beneath the nasal bone cephalically. (*E*) The spreader graft has been inserted between the left ULC and the septum. (*F*) Bilateral spreader grafts have been placed.

Complications of spreader grafts include the cephalic edge rotating anteriorly and becoming visible at the bony-cartilaginous junction, undercorrection with continued visible middle third collapse, and poor lateralization of the ULC with continued internal nasal valve stenosis. Tapering the cephalic edge of the spreader graft and inserting it beneath the nasal bone will lock it in place and prevent postoperative anterior rotation. Overcorrecting middle third depressions is often needed to adequately correct concavities there. Experienced surgeons are relying less on spreader grafts to correct internal nasal valve problems, adding batten grafts for greater stability and support of the internal nasal valve area posteriorly. Spreader grafts are most useful for correcting visible concavities and preventing unsightly inverted-V deformities and less useful for correcting internal nasal valve functional deficits (**Figs. 2–4**).

Flaring sutures, known as "Park sutures" after Dr. Stephen Park, are sometimes used to widen the internal nasal valve angle.[13] A horizontal mattress suture extends from the caudal/lateral area of the ULC, across the septum dorsum, and fixed to the contralateral ULC. The septum acts as a fulcrum when the suture is tightened, flaring the ULC laterally to increase the angle between the septum and ULC.[13] An alternative

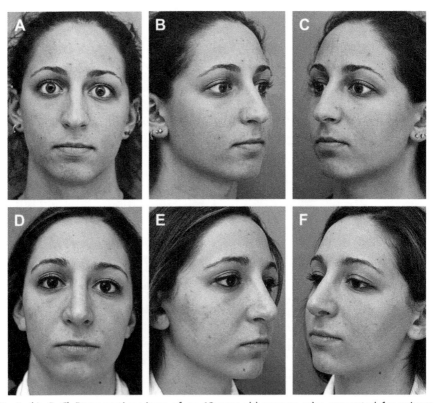

Fig. 2. (*A, B, C*) Preoperative views of an 18 year-old woman who presented for primary rhinoplasty. Note the pre-existing, inverted, V deformity and the exaggerated diamond shape of the nasion. Spreader grafts are needed to prevent postoperative collapse of her long ULC. (*D, E, F*) 2-year postoperative views. Surgery included dorsal reduction, bilateral lateral osteotomies, bilateral spreader grafts, dome-binding sutures, tongue-in-groove for medial crural support, and bilateral rim grafts. Observe the excellent stability of the middle-third with smooth, brow-tip lines bilaterally.

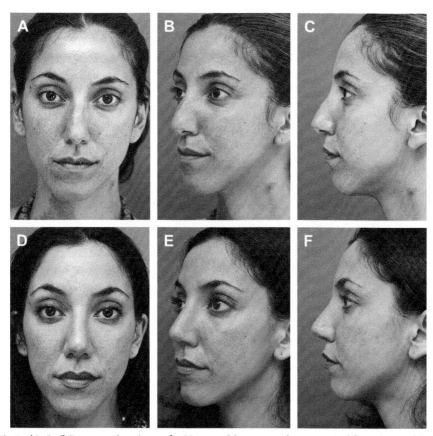

Fig. 3. (*A, B, C*) Preoperative views of a 29 year-old woman who presented for primary rhinoplasty. Note the moderate dorsal deviation to the right, with a collapsed left ULC. (*D, E, F*) 1-year postoperative views following rhinoplasty, including bilateral medial and lateral osteotomies, caudal septal shortening, left spreader graft, bilateral cephalic trims with dome-binding sutures and a columellar strut for medial crural support. Excellent symmetry and stability were achieved with the left spreader graft.

to the flaring suture is the suspension suture where a small incision, 1 cm anterior and inferior to the medial canthus, is made over the nasal bone to pass a suture under the superficial musculoaponeurotic system.[14] A separate endonasal intercartilaginous incision is made so that the suture can be passed around the ULC and directed back to the external nasal incision. Tightening of this suture results in lateralization and suspension of the ULC and thus increasing the nasal valve area.

Butterfly grafts are additional alternatives to widen the internal nasal valve.[15] These grafts use the intrinsic curvature of conchal cartilage and can be placed endonasally or by way of an open approach at the scroll area between the ULC and LLC to widen the internal nasal valve angle. Grafts are sutured in place with the caudal border of the graft deep to the cephalic border of the lateral crura. However, butterfly grafts have a higher tendency to alter cosmetic appearance by widening the nasal supratip region.

An alternative to the butterfly graft is a striated septal cartilage graft that can help open the internal valve. This graft is an excellent alternative as long as the supratip septum is slightly saddled so the graft blends well with the surrounding dorsum (**Fig. 5**).

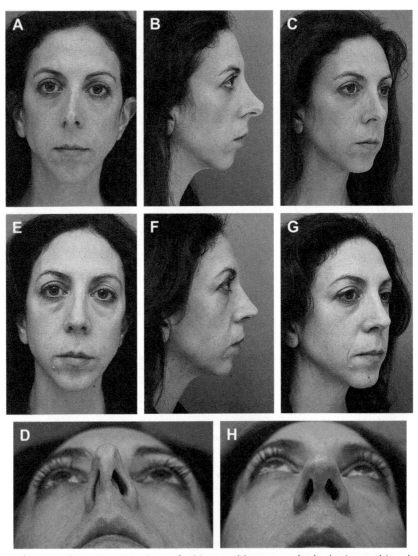

Fig. 4. (*A, B, C, D*) Preoperative views of a 39 year-old woman who had primary rhinoplasty 16 years prior, now with severe right-greater-than-left nasal obstruction. The dorsal septum is deviated right and ULC are collapsed. She also is overprojected with narrow nostrils, with the external nasal valve closed caused by the caudal septal deviation to the right. (*E, F, G, H*) 2-year postoperative views demonstrate excellent middle-third stability after bilateral spreader grafts. Vertical lobule division with cartilage overlap reduced her projection. Crushed cartilage camouflaged the open-roof deformity. Osteotomies were not performed. Other than a columellar strut, no additional grafting was required for the largely-intact lower-lateral cartilages.

The splay graft, described by Guyuron and colleagues,[16] is another technique where a conchal cartilage graft is placed in a pocket between the ULC and the underlying mucosa once the ULC is separated from the cartilaginous septum. The resulting T formation widens the internal valve angle and prevents collapse. A modified splay

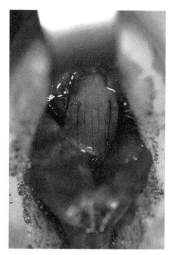

Fig. 5. The septal cartilage graft is striated longitudinally to break the surface spring enough for the graft to bend, but without losing its inherent recoil. When the graft is sutured across the dorsum with a horizontal mattress suture onto the underlying ULC, it flares them out and opens the internal nasal valves. The graft works best when there is a slight saddle, in this case from a previous septoplasty.

graft, described recently by Islam and colleagues,[17] has a few differences that may facilitate the operation, namely an endonasal approach, preservation of the ULC and septal cartilage junction, preservation of perichondrium on one side of the graft, thus with the potential possibility of decreasing duration, complications, and morbidity of the surgery.

Recently, the Monarch adjustable implant (Hanson Medical, Kingston, Washington) was approved by the Federal Drug Administration for the correction of nasal valve dysfunction, particularly in patients with nasal changes related to aging. This implant is designed to function essentially like a cartilaginous butterfly graft or effectively like an adjustable implanted Breathe-Right dilator (CNS Inc.). The Monarch implant is a dual material device made of an expanded polytetrafluoroethylene or reinforced silicone outer casing surrounding a malleable titanium core. The malleability of the device allows precise adjustments to obtain an optimal valve area with aesthetic balance. These adjustments can be made during, or after, surgery in the office setting. A recent follow-up study by Hurbis[18] demonstrated significant improvement in daytime snoring and nighttime nasal airway ratings on questionnaire data at 1 month after surgery, with slight improvement in questionnaire ratings at 6 months after surgery. Rhinometry data revealed increased static nasal valve area at 1 and 6 months after surgery, with minimal or no adverse effects.

While Z-plasty has been successfully described for correcting external nasal valve stenosis and cleft nasal deformity, intranasal Z-plasty for internal nasal valve narrowing is a novel technique. Dutton and Neidich[19] reported 12 subjects that underwent intranasal Z-plasty to correct narrowing of the nasal valve using triangular flaps to lateralize and lengthen the scroll region. These patients all had improvement in their subjective nasal valve obstruction and valve angle widening on nasal endoscopy. Flap mobilization can create mild cephalic alar rotation, further improving airflow. However, this series did not show any significant cosmetic deformity caused by this cephalic rotation.

SURGICAL MANAGEMENT OF THE EXTERNAL NASAL VALVE

The external nasal valve is composed primarily of the lateral crus of the LLC and is most commonly disturbed in aggressive alar cartilage reduction during rhinoplasty. The mainstay of surgical treatment of external valve collapse has been alar batten grafts.[13] Alar batten grafts augment weak or absent LLC, which may be congenital or secondary to prior rhinoplasty involving overaggressive cartilage resection during tip-modeling procedures. Septal or conchal cartilage can serve as sources for graft material. The graft should be long enough to be seated in the soft-tissue pocket starting at the level of the supra-alar crease, at the junction of the ULC and LLC, and extend over the bony pyriform aperture. For optimal cosmetic appearance, these grafts should be thin with beveled edges, and for maximal structural support, should be

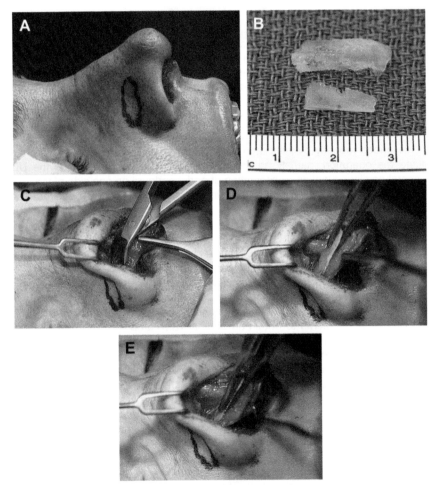

Fig. 6. Alar batten grafts. (*A*) The area of maximal weakness has been marked preoperatively. (*B*) Typical size of a batten graft (*top*). The graft ideally extends laterally onto the pyriform aperture for maximal stabilization of the lateral-nasal wall. (*C*) Pocket to receive graft being dissected with the tip scissors. (*D*) Graft being inserted into pocket. (*E*) Graft in position, before being suture-secured to underlying lateral crus.

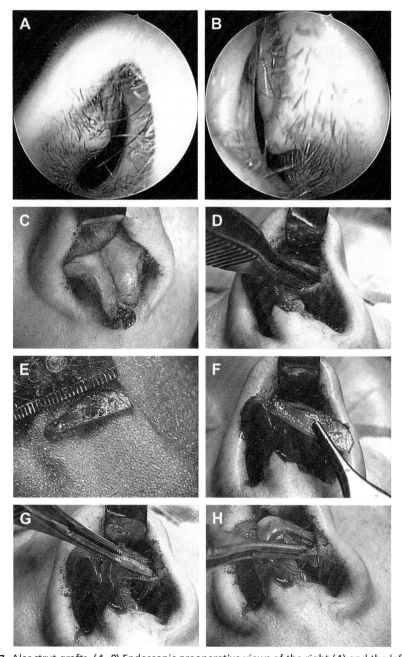

Fig. 7. Alar strut grafts. (*A, B*) Endoscopic preoperative views of the right (*A*) and the left (*B*) lateral crura of a patient who had undergone previous rhinoplasty. (*C*) Intraoperative view of the same patient, revealing a markedly over-resected right lateral crus and a largely intact but inwardly prolapsing left lateral crus. (*D*) The vestibular mucosa has been raised off the undersurface of the left lateral crus and a pocket has been created to receive an alar strut graft. (*E*) Typical size of an alar strut graft is 2 cm or longer. (*F, G, H*) The strut graft being placed into its pocket. It will be suture-secured to the overlying lateral crus.

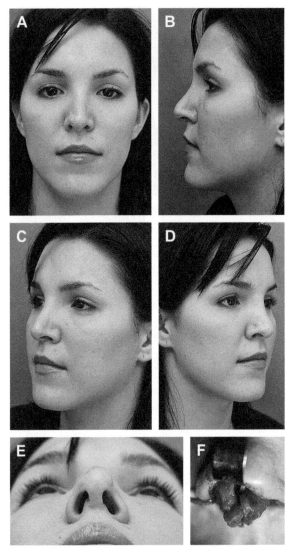

Fig. 8. (*A, B, C, D, E*) Preoperative views of a 23 year-old woman who had primary rhinoplasty 5 years prior. In addition to the scarred soft tip skin on the right, she has bilateral internal and external nasal valve stenosis. The polly beak is from scar. (*F*) Intraoperative view showing the massively weakened and distorted alar cartilages. Surgery included bilateral lateral osteotomies, excision of the scar from the supratip that was then wrapped round crushed cartilage and used to augment the upper third, bilateral spreader grafts, left alar batten and right alar strut grafts, and a columellar strut graft. (*G, H, I, J, K*). 2-year postoperative views demonstrating good symmetry and stability of the nose. The internal and external nasal valves are strong and widely patent.

wider laterally along the pyriform aperture. The exact size and placement of the batten grafts depend on the specific individual deformities, but should primarily reinforce those areas of the alar lobule which collapse with inspiration, without changing the resting position of the valve. Battens may be fixed in place with either a transcutaneous

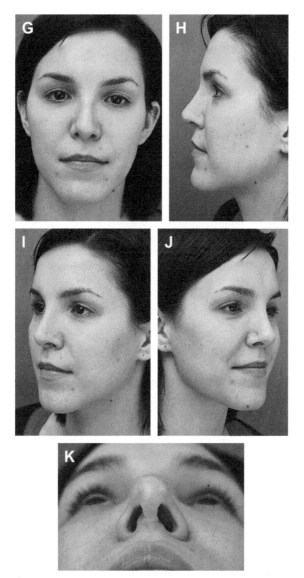

Fig. 8. (*continued*)

or transmucosal resorbable suture to fix the batten graft in its pocket. If carefully placed and tapered, alar batten grafts need not create fullness at the site of the graft. If filling is desired, the graft can be contoured appropriately for optimal results (**Fig. 6**).

Toriumi and colleagues[20] described their experience with alar batten grafts in 46 subjects and found that all but one had marked improvement in nasal airway obstruction. Postoperative examinations revealed significant increases in internal or external nasal valve with increased structural support and patency of the external valve upon moderate-to-deep inspiration. They concluded that alar batten grafts are effective techniques for long-term correction of nasal valve collapse in properly selected patients without intranasal scarring, loss of vestibular skin, or excessive narrowing of the pyriform aperture.

An alternative to alar batten grafts that overlay the lateral crura are alar strut grafts that underlay the lateral crura. They provide support to the external nasal valve or the internal nasal valve, depending upon their positioning. The graft is placed by elevating the vestibular skin off the undersurface of the lateral crus. The graft is usually directed more caudally than the posterior portion of the lateral crus, essentially acting as an alar batten in the region of the external valve devoid of cartilage. Its medial portion, therefore, supports the lateral crus, lateral to the dome, while its lateral portion supports the hinge area, where ligaments course from the lateral crus toward the pyriform aperture. Indications for the alar strut graft include inward curvature of the lateral crus, double-convex lateral crus, and weak lateral crus. Alar strut grafts are also helpful when transposing cephalically-oriented lateral crura to help stabilize them once they have been translocated more caudally (**Figs. 7** and **8**).

Another technique for correcting a flaccid external nasal valve is the lateral crus pull-up described by Menger,[21] where the lateral crus of the LLC is rotated in a supero-lateral direction and held in place with a permanent spanning suture through the pyriform aperture. This technique involves dissection through an intercartilaginous incision toward the caudal border of the bony pyramid. Once the soft-tissue envelope, including the periosteum, is elevated, a small hole is drilled in the bony pyriform aperture at the desired location. Menger recommends using a Gore-Tex (WL Gore & Associates Inc., Newark, Delaware) suture given its strength and decreased chance of cutting through cartilage over time.

Cicatricial stenosis of the external nasal valve can be corrected with a number of surgical techniques, including Z-plasty, skin grafts, alar interposition, and composite grafts. Small webs may be divided primarily and then stented.

External nasal valve obstruction caused by tip ptosis is either caused by soft tissue ptosis, resulting from bulky excess tissue, or structural ptosis, resulting from cartilaginous, ligamentous, or muscular deficiencies in tip support.[9] Idiopathic tip soft-tissue bulk is usually associated with thick redundant skin and subcutaneous tissue in the supratip region, which can be excised to relieve soft-tissue bulk. Structural ptosis can result from weakened support from the medial crura or columella, and may require a tip-lifting maneuver where a horizontal mattress suture is placed from the LLC to the periosteum of the nasal bones.

Dynamic external nasal valve dysfunction can also occur because of decreased nasal muscular tone secondary to facial paralysis or aging, resulting in cartilaginous and soft-tissue laxity. This may require a combination of a tip-lifting maneuver and soft-tissue excision. In cases of severe facial paralysis, patients who undergo nerve grafts, cranial nerve XII to VII anastomosis, or VII to VII crossover for facial reanimation, may regain little or some of their nasal valve tone. However, this does not occur in many cases, and these patients often benefit from additional nasal valve reconstruction. A retrospective review by Soler and colleagues[22] examined 28 subjects undergoing facial nerve resection as part of their oncologic ablative surgery and found that those patients who received immediate nasal valve suspension reconstruction, using a suture-suspension technique to secure the nasal valve to the inferior orbital rim periosteum at the time of ablation, had significantly fewer symptoms of nasal obstruction than the control group who did not undergo immediate reconstruction. These authors suggest that the nasal valve should be addressed at the time of initial facial nerve resection for optimal outcomes.

Paradoxical lateral crura are a relatively uncommon phenomenon where the curvature of the lateral crus is reversed and concave rather than convex. A lateral crura flip-flop procedure can be beneficial in these patients, where the paradoxical portion of the lateral crura is resected, flipped over, and sutured back into place to resemble normal LLC curvature (**Fig. 9**). If further external nasal valve support is needed to overcome collapse during inspiration, then alar batten or tip grafts may be needed.

OUTCOMES OF FUNCTIONAL RHINOPLASTY

Interest in outcomes analysis after functional rhinoplasty has been increasing in recent years to assess the efficacy of functional rhinoplasty techniques.[1,23–28] Quantitative measurement of the effects of surgery has been around for some time, including nasal peak inspiratory flow and acoustic rhinometry, and qualitative measurements by way of retrospective patient questionnaires. In 1996, Constantinides, Adamson, and Cole[23] proved that spreader grafts reduce nasal resistance to airflow using posterior rhinomanometry. More recently, validated measurement tools, such as the Nasal Obstruction Symptoms Evaluation (NOSE) scale, have been developed. A prospective

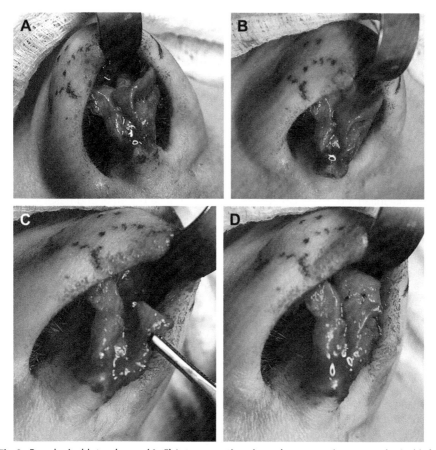

Fig. 9. Paradoxical lateral crus. (*A, B*) Intraoperative views demonstrating a paradoxical left-lateral crus. See the severe concavity in the longitudinal and transverse planes. (*C*) The lateral crus has been removed. All that remains is the left dome. (*D*) The lateral crus has been flipped over, replaced and sutured to the left dome. The previous concavity is now a convexity, symmetric with the contralateral side (not shown).

observational outcomes study on subjects who underwent functional rhinoplasty examined preoperative and postoperative NOSE scores and found that all subjects demonstrated significant airway improvement in all subcategories based on the specific procedure that was performed.[25] Additionally, a large recent meta-analysis by Rhee and colleagues[24] reviewed the efficacy of functional rhinoplasty techniques for the treatment of nasal valve dysfunction over the past 25 years found that there is substantial level 4 evidence (case series) to support the efficacy of current functional rhinoplasty techniques. The authors suggest a need for increased use of comparison cohorts and standardized objective outcome measures to strengthen evidence supporting what is already recognized clinically.

SUMMARY

Treatment of the nasal valve, both surgical and nonsurgical, continues to improve with better understanding of nasal anatomy and physiology and advancements in technology.

While spreader grafts and alar batten grafts have been the mainstay of treatment of nasal valve dysfunction for quite some time, newer techniques are emerging and gaining popularity among surgeons. Areas for future improvements include better use of standardized-outcome assessments to evaluate efficacy of specific surgical procedures in repairing nasal valve abnormalities. Nasal anatomy and physiology is unique across individuals, and nasal valve dysfunction should always be treated with a tailored regimen specific to the individual deformities.

REFERENCES

1. Rhee J, Poetker D, Smith TL, et al. Nasal valve surgery improves disease specific quality of life. Laryngoscope 2005;115:437–40.
2. Mink PJ. Le nez comme voie respiratorie. Presse Otolaryngol (Belg) 1903;481–96 [French].
3. Constantian MB, Brian CR. The relative importance of septal and nasal valvular surgery in correcting airway obstruction in primary and secondary rhinoplasty. Plast Reconstr Surg 1996;98(1):38–54.
4. Miman MC, Deliktas H, Ozturan O, et al. Internal nasal valve: revisited with objective facts. Otolaryngol Head Neck Surg 2006;134(1):41–7.
5. Kern EB, Wang TD. Nasal valve surgery. In: Daniel RK, Regnault P, Goldwyn RM, editors. Aesthetic plastic surgery: rhinoplasty. London: Little, Brown and Co.; 1993. p. 613–30.
6. Grymer LF. Reduction rhinoplasty and nasal patency: change in the cross-sectional area of the nose evaluated by acoustic rhinometry. Laryngoscope 1995;105:429–31.
7. Khosh JM, Jen A, Honrado C, et al. Nasal valve reconstruction: experience in 53 consecutive patients. Arch Facial Plast Surg 2004;6:167–71.
8. Sheen JH. Spreader graft: a method of reconstructing the roof of the middle nasal vault following rhinoplasty. Plast Reconstr Surg 1984;73(2):230–7.
9. Schlosser RJ, Park SS. Functional rhinoplasty. Otolaryngol Clin North Am 1999; 32(1):37–51.
10. Constantinides MS, Galli SK, Miller PJ. A simple and reliable method of patient evaluation in the surgical treatment of nasal obstruction. Ear Nose Throat J 2002;81(10):734–7.
11. Nyte CP. Hyaluronic acid spreader-graft injection for internal nasal valve collapse. Ear Nose Throat J 2007;86(5):272–3.

12. Inanli S, Sari M, Yazici MZ. The results of concurrent functional endoscopic sinus surgery and rhinoplasty. J Craniofac Surg 2008;19(3):701–4.
13. Ballert JA, Park SS. Functional rhinoplasty: treatment of the dysfunctional nasal sidewall. Facial Plast Surg 2006;22(1):49–54.
14. Nuara MJ, Mobley SR. Nasal valve suspension revisited. Laryngoscope 2007; 117:2100–6.
15. Clark JM, Cook TA. The 'butterfly' graft in functional secondary rhinoplasty. Laryngoscope 2002;112:1917–25.
16. Guyuron B, Michelow BJ, Englebardt C. Upper lateral splay graft. Plast Reconstr Surg 1998;102:2169–77.
17. Islam A, Arslan N, Felek SA, et al. Reconstruction of the internal nasal valve: modified splay graft technique with endonasal approach. Laryngoscope 2008; 118:1739–43.
18. Hurbis CG. A follow-up study of the Monarch adjustable implant for correction of nasal valve dysfunction. Arch Facial Plast Surg 2008;10(2):142–3.
19. Dutton JM, Neidich MJ. Intranasal Z-plasty for internal nasal valve collapse. Arch Facial Plast Surg 2008;10(3):164–8.
20. Toriumi DM, Josen J, Weinberger M, et al. Use of alar batten grafts for correction of nasal valve collapse. Arch Otolaryngol Head Neck Surg 1997;123(8):802–8.
21. Menger DJ. Lateral crus pull-up: a method for collapse of the external nasal valve. Arch Facial Plast Surg 2006;8(5):333–7.
22. Soler ZM, Rosenthal E, Wax MK. Immediate nasal valve reconstruction after facial nerve resection. Arch Facial Plast Surg 2008;10(5):312–5.
23. Constantinides MS, Adamson PA, Cole P. The long term effects of open cosmetic septorhinoplasty on nasal air flow. Arch Otolaryngol Head Neck Surg 1996;122: 41–5.
24. Rhee JS, Arganbright JM, McMullin BT, et al. Evidence supporting functional rhinoplasty or nasal valve repair: a 25-year systematic review. Otolaryngol Head Neck Surg 2008;139(1):10–20.
25. Most SP. Analysis of outcomes after functional rhinoplasty using a disease-specific quality-of-life instrument. Arch Facial Plast Surg 2006;8(5):306–9.
26. Costa F, Robiony M, Salvo I, et al. Simultaneous functional endoscopic sinus surgery and esthetic rhinoplasty in orthognathic patients. J Oral Maxillofac Surg 2008;66(7):1370–7.
27. Faris C, Koury E, Kothari P, et al. Functional rhinoplasty with batten and spreader grafts for correction of internal nasal valve incompetence. Rhinology 2006;44(2): 114–7.
28. Fischer H, Gubisch W. Nasal valves – importance and surgical procedures. Facial Plast Surg 2006;22:266–80.

Open Septoplasty: Indications and Treatment

Mohamad Chaaban, MD[a], Anil R. Shah, MD[b,*]

KEYWORDS
- Open septoplasty • Deviated nasal septum
- Rhinoplasty • Septal repair • Septal surgery
- Nasal obstruction • Septoplasty surgery

HISTORY

Open septoplasty is the use of open rhinoplasty approach to address the septum. Open rhinoplasty's history is long. Open rhinoplasty probably first started in 600 BC when Sushutra and Samhita practiced in India.[1] The first transcolumellar incision approach to the nasal tip was described by Rethi from Budapest in 1921. He described a method of using a high transverse columellar incision that joins two marginal incisions.[2] Rethi did not extend the incision to expose the whole nasal pyramid. His idea was not accepted because of the easier utility of the subcutaneous operation on the nasal tips. Sercer of Zagreb in 1956[3] extended the incision and described what was known at that time as "decortication" of the nose and defined it as a temporary separation of the nasal skin from the nasal pyramid.

Although the earlier manifestations of open rhinoplasty were used to address nasal tip deformities, Padovan, Sercer's successor at Zagreb[3] was the first to describe the utility of the open approach to the septum. Goodman in 1973 made the open approach to the nose more systematic and expanded on the indications and included the combined external deformities of the nose and the septum as one of the indications. Andersen and Wright are generally credited with popularizing open rhinoplasty and its use with open septoplasty techniques.[4]

ANATOMY

The nasal septum is composed of cartilaginous and bony parts (**Fig. 1**). The bones that make up the septum are the perpendicular plate of the ethmoid bone posterosuperiorly and the vomer, together with the crests of the maxillary and palatine bones,

[a] Department of Otolaryngology, Head and Neck Surgery, University of Chicago Hospitals, 5841 S Maryland Avenue E-102, Chicago, IL 60637, USA
[b] Division of Facial Plastic Surgery, Department of Otolaryngology-Head and Neck Surgery, University of Chicago, 845 N. Michigan Avenue, Suite 934, E. Chicago, IL 60611, USA
* Corresponding author.
E-mail address: shah@shahfacialplastics.com (A.R. Shah).

Otolaryngol Clin N Am 42 (2009) 513–519
doi:10.1016/j.otc.2009.03.012

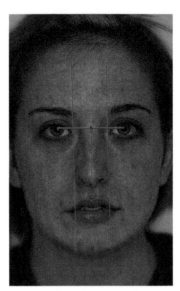

Fig. 1. A nasal symmetry grid is created by drawing a line connecting the pupils as well as two lines perpendicular to the Frankfort Horizontal line from the medial canthus. Several points are then placed including: (*Point A*) central portion of pupil line; (*Point B*) subnasale; (*Point C*) philtrum of upper lip; (*Point D*) midportion of chin. To determine, nasal symmetry, a line is connected from *Point A* to *Point B*.

posteroinferiorly. The perpendicular plate of the ethmoid unites superiorly with the cribriform plate and anterosuperiorly with the frontal and nasal bones. The vomer articulates superiorly with the sphenoid and the perpendicular plate of ethmoid; and inferiorly with the maxillary and palatine crests.

The septal cartilage comes in contact with both the perpendicular plates of ethmoid and the vomer posteriorly and the maxillary bone inferiorly. The septal cartilage itself has an anterior, middle, and posterior septal angle, which relates to the nasal tip and its support. The relationship between the fibrous attachments of the septum and lower lateral cartilages clearly impact the support and projection of the nose.

The septum may play a larger role in nasal tip support than previously described. A study by the senior author (ARS) suggests that even routine septoplasty maneuvers can lead to loss of nasal tip support. Advanced septoplasty maneuvers are more likely to impact the projection of the nose. Therefore, surgeons should have the ability to either maintain or adjust nasal tip projection if necessary, especially with more advanced techniques described here.

PHYSIOLOGY

In the normal nose, the maximal airflow is through the middle meatus. Poiseuille's law states that the laminar flow of a gas in a tube is inversely proportional to one half of its diameter to the fourth power. Although the nasal flow in the nose is turbulent, the law is generally applicable. For this reason, the primary determinant of the nasal airflow is the minimal cross-sectional area of the nasal cavity, which is well determined to be the internal nasal valve. The internal nasal valve is defined by the area created by the junction of the nasal septum and the upper lateral nasal cartilages. Narrowing of this area by an anterior septal deviation or high dorsal deflection will thus create high resistance in the nasal airway.

Changes to the angle of the internal nasal valve, which is normally between 15–20 degrees, alters airflow and subsequently causes obstruction. Causes of obstruction include but are not limited to: wide or deviated nasal septum, collapse of the internal nasal valve, tip ptosis, and loss of the upper lateral cartilages.[5] It has been shown that correcting the septum, together with the internal nasal valve, helps in improving airflow flow five times than when compared with correcting the septum alone.[6]

Open septoplasty provides an excellent exposure to the internal nasal valve, nasal tip and the cartilaginous and bony vaults. It has been shown that the point of maximum thickness of the septum is at the anteriosuperior angle.[6]

DIAGNOSIS

One of challenges of the surgeon is diagnosing the septal deflection. Anterior rhinoscopy alone is inadequate means of determining the severity of the deviated septum. A combination of skills is necessary to accurately diagnose a severely deviated septum including visualization, palpation, and endoscopy.

The diagnosis of septal deviations begins with taking an adequate history from the patient. This history should include a history of trauma to the nose, nasal airway problems, and prior nasal surgeries.

Visualization of the external appearance of the nose is vital. On frontal view, a deviated septum will sometimes manifest with an external deviation. Standardized photography will allow for accurate digital measures to be performed. When taking the frontal view photograph, the authors suggest that the patient's head be calibrated with Frankfort horizontal line, including lining up the external auditory canals to be parallel to the horizon line.

The senior author (ARS) has developed a method of distinguishing facial asymmetry from nasal asymmetry. He finds it is imperative not only identify asymmetry within the nose, but how it relates to the face. First, a line is drawn from pupil to pupil. Two lines perpendicular to this line are drawn from the medial canthus inferiorly. A measured point is created at the exact middistance between the pupils (Point A). Additional points are created at the subnasale (Point B), phitrum of the lip (Point C), and midline of the chin (Point D). A line is created by joining Point A and Point B to determine the nasal asymmetry.

Deviation of the nose can be compared on either side of this line. Further evaluation of the nose can be seen by dividing the nose into thirds by placing lines dividing the nasal bones from the middle vault and middle vault from the nasal tip. This evaluation can be useful in distinguishing bony deviation from middle vault and septal deviation (see **Fig. 1**; **Fig. 2**).

A perfectly straight nose on an asymmetric face will not appear symmetric. The nose must relate to the face. To help determine facial symmetry an additional line can be created by connecting Point A to the line which bisects Point B and Point C. The nose will appear to fit with the face if it relates to this line rather than a line perpendicular to the Frankfort horizontal line.

The baseview of the nose can also reveal information regarding the degree of deviation in the nose. A deviated columella often correlates to a deviated septum. In addition, a footplate seen comprising the airway will often correlate to a deviated septum lateralizing the footplate.

Anterior rhinoscopy is important to allow for visualization of the septum and its relationship to the remainder of the nose. However, there are recognized limits of anterior rhinoscopy. Endoscopy can be helpful to visualize the posterior aspect of the septum and more precise visualization of the internal nasal valve.

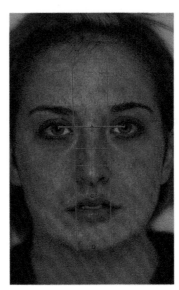

Fig. 2. Asymmetries within each portion of the nose can be seen by dividing: the bony portion from the middle vault; and middle vault from nasal tip.

Visualization alone is not sufficient to diagnose the degree of septal deviation. Palpation of the anterior septal angle, middle septal, and posterior septal angle will help to determine the type of caudal septal deflection. In particular, the posterior septal angle may or may not be fixed to the nasal spine or maxilla. Also, the nasal tip should be balloted to help determine how significant the nasal tip strength.

TECHNIQUE OPEN SEPTOPLASTY

The operation is typically performed under either general anesthesia or intravenous sedation. The authors prefer the use of general anesthesia because of the airway protection provided by an endotracheal tube. If general anesthesia is used, then injections of 1% lidocaine with epinephrine 1:100,000 are performed at the level of the glabella, columella, nasolabial fold and the septum.[3] Hydrodissection plays a critical component in septoplasty and the surgeon should see a whitish blanch as well as note separation of the mucoperichondrial flap from the underlying septum. The authors use topical Afrin on pledgets after injection for further vasoconstriction of the mucoperichondrial tissues.

First an inverted V-shaped incision with a no. 11 blade is fashioned on the columella. The superior aspect of the incision should always be below the apex of the nostril and typically begin at the narrowest portion of the columella. A marginal incision is made with a 15 blade along the caudal edge of the alar cartilages. The location of the caudal edge usually is at the cephalic boundary of the hair-carrying portion of the vestibule.[3] In revision rhinoplasty, patients with "soft lower lateral cartilages" determination of the caudal edge may not be straightforward. In these instances, the surgeon can avoid the marginal incision and dissect on top of the lower lateral cartilages in an incremental fashion.

With the use of the skin hooks and converse scissors, the nasal tip skin is elevated off the columellar infrastructure. Care is taken to keep the thin skin over the medial crura intact. The dissection is continued to over the nasal tip where the nasal tip is lifted with a two-pronged hook and later by the ala protector with lip. This dissection is performed starting medially and then moving laterally. The soft tissue envelope is lifted up in the subperichondrial plane, which reduces bleeding and enhances healing.

Exposure of the septum can take place in a variety of methods depending on the location of the deviation. In cases where the nasolabial angle will be altered, significant changes in projection, large septal deflections within the nose and in anterior septal deflections, dissection takes place between the medial crus. Here the fibrous attachments of the medial crus are separated until the anterior septal angle is identified. This is the most common method of accessing septal deflections. In cases where there is only a dorsal deflection, dissection of the septum can take place by separating the upper lateral cartilages and placing spreader grafts. This indication is rather limited and seldom incorporated. In cases where the septal deflection is located within the central portion of the cartilage, exposure can take place from a hemitransfixion or Kilian incision. The robust blood supply of the nose allows for separate Kilian incision to be made even in open rhinoplasty.

Specific Indications and Applications of Open Septoplasty

Some authors feel that open septoplasty allows the surgeon to have a better look at the osseocartilaginous framework of which deformities can be accurately diagnosed.[4] The authors contend that a thorough physical examination will allow for accurate diagnosis of septal deviation and deformity and that open septoplasty is not to be used for diagnosis. In addition, there is not a hard-set rule of when a nose should be opened under any circumstances, including for a septal deflection.

A severely deviated anterior septum located within the anterior 2 cm of the caudal septum is typically a reason enough to open a nose. A noticeable exception to a deviated deflection here would be a straight caudal deflection, which may be more amenable to being repositioned via swinging door technique. Many anterior septal deflections can be repaired by repositioning the septal cartilage and securing it to the periosteum of the nasal spine. Cartilaginous deflections with a significant concavity or convexity may require excision and replacement of this component. Disarticulation and repair of the entire septum, although necessary in some instances, may require large amounts of cartilage but should only be performed in select cases.

Another indication for open septoplasty is the deviated dorsal septum. Here, a variety of maneuvers can be performed in order to straighten the dorsal component. Sometimes, a unilateral spreader graft, placed on the concave surface, can assist in providing enough strength to help straighten the septum. Other times, asymmetric spreader grafts may be required to provide further strength. For even more dramatic deviations, an excision and replacement of the deviated component may be necessary to provide sufficient correction of the deviation.

Patients with "short" nasal septums often benefit from extension of the existing septum. One maneuver, which can extend a septum, is the caudal extension graft. It can be used to adjust septal rotation and projection to help contribute to the position of the nasal tip. In patients with a poorly projected nasal tip, often times open septoplasty is necessary to allow for sufficient manipulation of the tip position to adequately project the nose. Some patients with poorly projected noses will have a ptotic nose as well. These patients may notice improvement in breathing with restoration of the nose with a more obtuse nasolabial angle.

The significantly deviated septum may require near total excision of the deviated septum and reconstruction. Although some authors remove the entire septum, the authors of this article contend that maintaining a small cartilaginous attachment to the bony septum is a safer and more effective means of repairing septal deviations.

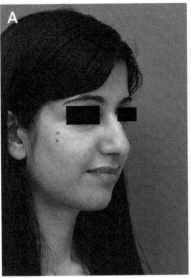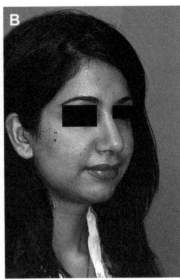

Fig. 3. Patient with intraoperative separation of bony cartilaginous junction. Her nasal profile was preserved by connecting supporting the middle third of the nose through drill holes created in the nasal bones. In addition, soft tissue onlay at bony cartilaginous junction is placed to ensure a smooth dorsum long term. Patient seen preoperatively (*A*) and postoperatively (*B*), with smooth dorsal profile at 1-year postoperative visit.

Attaching cartilaginous elements to bony elements is difficult and can lead to slight shifts in reapproximation, while attaching cartilage to an existing piece of cartilage can lead to improved overall stability.

Another reason for open septoplasty is complete separation of the bony and cartilaginous components of the septum. In this case, the cartilagionous elements of the nose must be reapproximated to the bony elements of the nose. A previous author described a classification system to help identify and repair entire separation of the bony cartilaginous septum.[5] The senior author believes this state is under diagnosed and has identified six cases of complete disarticulation of the bony cartilagionus septum. The repair consists of drilling holes through the bony septum, placement of bilateral spreader grafts, and a soft augmentation graft over the bony cartilagionous septum. This is important as the connection between the cartilage and bone may create a small depression less than 1 mm at one year and requires soft tissue camouflage (**Fig. 3**).

SUMMARY

Open septoplasty represents a powerful approach to septal deflections. Septoplasty is the critical foundation of rhinoplasty and functional improvement in the nose. Judicious use of open septoplasty and incorporation of advanced septoplasty maneuvers may help improve septal deflections.

REFERENCES

1. Mc Dowell F. Ancient ear lobe and rhinoplastic operations in India (from Sushruta Samhita). In: The source book of plastic surgery. Baltimore (MD): Williams Wilkins Cy; 1977.

2. Rethi A. Operation to shorten an excessively long nose. Rev Chir Plast 1934;2: 85–7.
3. Mangat DS, Smith BJ. Septoplasty via the open approach. Facial Plast Surg 1988; 5(2):161–6.
4. Gunter JP. The merits of the open approach in rhinoplasty. Plast Reconstr Surg 1997;99(3):863–7.
5. Gunter M. Surgery of the nasal septum. Semin Plast Surg 2006;22(4):223–9.
6. Ashmit G, Gupta A, Brooks D, et al. Surgical access to the internal nasal valve. Arch Facial Plast Surg 2003;5:155–8.

Congenital Nasal Pyriform Aperture Stenosis

James R. Tate, MD, Jonathan Sykes, MD, FACS*

KEYWORDS

• Stenosis • Nasal • Pyriform • Congenital • Pediatric • Airway

Congenital nasal pyriform aperture stenosis (CNPAS) is a rare cause of nasal obstruction in neonates. It is caused by a bony overgrowth of the medial nasal process of the maxilla. In their landmark article in 1989, Brown and colleagues[1] first clinically described this condition. In their series of six patients, they suggested that this condition arose as an isolated anomaly. In 1992, Arlis and Ward[2] described a series of six patients who had CNPAS, four of whom had evidence of associated anomalies. Since that time, approximately 30 cases have been described in the literature in the form of case reports and small case series.[3] It is now clear that pyriform aperture stenosis can occur in isolation or can be associated with other anomalies.[2] The true incidence of CNPAS is unknown, given the variable degrees of stenosis and clinical manifestations. When present, CNPAS is usually bilateral. CNPAS can easily be mistaken for choanal stenosis or even atresia, given the similar clinical presentation.

ANATOMY AND EMBRYOLOGY

The normal development of the lip and palate occurs during the embryonic period, which is the first 12 weeks of intrauterine development. Specifically, nasal development begins at approximately 3 weeks of gestation. The nasal development begins with the formation of paired olfactory nasal placodes that develop into nasal pits. The nasal pits gradually deepen to separate the frontonasal process into medial and lateral nasal processes. The paired medial processes fuse in the midline at approximately 4 to 7 weeks of gestation to form the primary palate. This fusion also forms the premaxilla, philtrum of the upper lip, columella, and nasal tip. The lateral processes eventually fuse with the maxilla to form the pyriform aperture and lateral nasal wall.[1] Secondary palate development begins after the primary palate is formed at approximately 8 weeks of gestation.

Facial Plastic and Reconstructive Surgery, Department of Otolaryngology, Head and Neck Surgery, University of California at Davis Medical Center, 2521 Stockton Boulevard, Suite 6206, Sacramento, CA 95817, USA
* Corresponding author.
E-mail address: jonathan.sykes@ucdmc.ucdavis.edu (J. Sykes).

Otolaryngol Clin N Am 42 (2009) 521–525
doi:10.1016/j.otc.2009.03.006
0030-6665/09/$ – see front matter © 2009 Elsevier Inc. All rights reserved.

oto.theclinics.com

The pyriform aperture is a pear-shaped bony inlet bounded by the nasal bone superiorly, the nasal process of the maxilla laterally, and the horizontal process inferiorly. The pyriform aperture is the narrowest most anterior bony portion of the nasal airway. Any decrease in cross-sectional area leads to a significant increase in nasal airway resistance and associated nasal airway obstruction.[4]

The developmental mechanism for formation of CNPAS remains unclear. Brown and colleagues[1] hypothesized that at 4 months of gestation, an overgrowth of maxillary ossification at the nasal process of maxilla leads to CNPAS (**Fig. 1**).

EVALUATION

The differential diagnosis for nasal obstruction in the infant is limited and should include septal displacement, nasopharyngeal mass, pyriform aperture stenosis, choanal stenosis, and atresia. It is important to remember that infants are obligate nasal breathers until the age of approximately 4 months. In those patients in whom there is difficulty passing a catheter by way of the nose, choanal stenosis and pyriform aperture stenosis should be included in the differential diagnosis.

Patients who have CNPAS typically present with evidence of nasal airway obstruction with cyclic cyanosis relieved by crying, similar to patients who have bilateral posterior choanal atresia.[1] Initial management centers on the establishment of an adequate airway, usually with an oral airway or McGovern nipple. In mild cases of obstruction with a stable airway and absence of feeding difficulties, conservative treatment is adequate. Conservative treatment consists of nasal humidification and decongestants with diligent follow-up. In severe cases, patients may require immediate intubation with ventilatory support. Ultimately, infants with severe nasal obstruction or congestion and difficulty in breathing have poor weight gain. These children are strong candidates for surgical intervention.

Although the diagnosis is often suggested by history and physical examination, radiographic confirmation should always be obtained. The radiographic imaging of choice is fine-cut CT with axial and coronal sections from the palate to the orbit. Intravenous contrast is usually not necessary. CT provides excellent bony detail, and therefore accurate analysis of the bony pyriform aperture and choanal anatomy. The finding of bony overgrowth of the nasal processes with resultant narrowing of nasal passages anteriorly confirms the diagnosis (**Fig. 2**).[1]

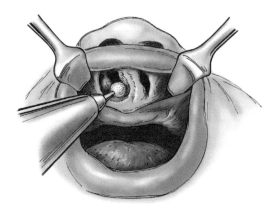

Fig. 1. Sublabial approach to the pyriform aperture. A drill is used to increase the cross-sectional area of the pyriform aperture.

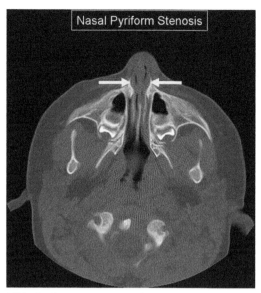

Fig. 2. CT scan of a child who has CNPAS. Note the inward bowing of the nasal processes of the maxillary bone with the pyriform aperture measuring 7 mm (*arrows*).

More recently, Lee and colleagues[5] have described the use of three-dimensional (3D) CT for the evaluation of CNPAS. These researchers suggested that using 3D CT gives a more precise evaluation of the amount of nasal process of the maxilla to be ablated, and therefore aids surgeons in the preoperative treatment planning and postoperative evaluations.

Patients who have CNPAS in association with a single central maxillary incisor should be further evaluated, because there may be an association with holoprosencephaly (HPE) (**Fig. 3**).

HPE is characterized by failure of the prosencephalon (forebrain) to divide into bilateral cerebral hemispheres, ultimately leading to defects in the development of the face. According to Levison and colleagues,[6] CNPAS can occur as a microform

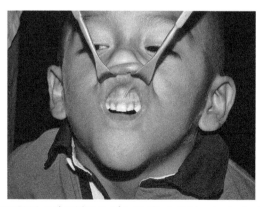

Fig. 3. Child who has CPAS and evidence of a single central megaincisor.

manifestation of the HPE spectrum, which includes a single maxillary central incisor. The more severe forms of HPE are usually fatal. The inheritance of HPE seems complex but may show evidence of autosomal dominant inheritance with variable expressivity. HPE has been associated with premaxillary dysgenesis. In fact, CNPAS has been reported to have an association with a single maxillary central incisor in up to 60% of cases.[7] Other midline defects associated with HPE include absent upper labial frenulum, microcephaly, midface hypoplasia, and cleft palate.[6] In such cases, chromosomal analysis and MRI to assess the hypothalamic-pituitary-thyroid-adrenal axis and brain are indicated.[2,8] Additionally, some investigators recommend an endocrinology workup and electrolyte evaluation.[4,9] Evaluation by means of a craniofacial panel, including a geneticist, should also be considered.

TREATMENT AND MANAGEMENT

The long-term data on the nonsurgical management of CNPAS are limited. In a report of two patients, Lee and colleagues[10] suggested that if patients are able to tolerate conservative management, their nasal airway is likely to improve with growth, typically within 6 months of birth. Some have suggested that the ability to pass a 5-French catheter accurately predicts the success of nonsurgical management.[11]

Surgical treatment is indicated in those patients with nasal obstruction associated with airway distress, unresponsiveness to conservative treatment, or poor weight gain. The timing of this intervention is controversial. In patients with a stable respiratory status, many surgeons apply the rule of "10s," in that surgery is deferred until the child reaches 10 lb, 10 weeks of age, or a hemoglobin rate of 10 mg/dL so as to operate on a larger and potentially more stable patient.[1,12]

The most used surgical approach is by means of a sublabial technique.[1] This approach has proved to be safe and effective. The patient is orally intubated, and the sublabial region infiltrated with Xylocaine 1% with 1:100,000 epinephrine for vasoconstriction. A sublabial incision is made, and the soft tissues and mucosa are elevated in a subperiosteal plane off the bony pyriform aperture. Great care is taken to avoid injury to the nasolacrimal ducts. Using diamond burrs and loupe magnification, the bony overgrowth is shaved down to widen the bony nasal inlet.[1,12] Occasionally, in patients with severe nasal obstruction, reduction of the inferior turbinates may also improve postoperative success. Although there have been no reliable standards for the size or length of time of postsurgical stenting, current standards call for enough width to pass a 3.5-mm endotracheal tube. Stents are typically left in place for 2 to 4 weeks.[1] Others have used the placement of soft silastic nasal stents (Dow Corning, Midland, Michigan) sutured to the columella for 5 to 7 days, with excellent results.[3] In the series of 14 patients treated in this manner by Losken and colleagues,[3] there were no cases of restenosis after a mean follow-up of 2.4 years. In any case, appropriate care for these stents with suctioning and saline irrigation needs to be diligently taught to the family before discharge.

An alternative surgical approach is by means of an endonasal technique. Although this approach may be possible in adults, it has proved to give inadequate visualization in infants.[1] Surgical risks include tooth bud damage, injury to the nasolacrimal ducts, and midfacial and nasal developmental hypoplasia.

SUMMARY

CNPAS is a rare cause of nasal obstruction in the neonate and has only been described as a clinical entity in the past 20 years. Initial evaluation should focus on the differentiation between choanal and pyriform aperture stenosis with a fine-cut

CT scan with axial and coronal views. CNPAS is often associated with other anomalies. If one suspects additional anomalies, a chromosome analysis and MRI scan are indicated. Surgical repair should be undertaken in those patients with respiratory difficulty or poor weight gain. In the infant, the sublabial approach is the most ideal. The bony aperture should be widened with great care to preserve nasal mucosa. Postoperative stenting aids in maintenance of the airway. This approach to treatment has proved to have a high degree of clinical success with minimal evidence of restenosis.

REFERENCES

1. Brown O, Myer C, Manning S. Congenital nasal pyriform aperture stenosis. Laryngoscope 1989;99:86–91.
2. Arlis H, Ward RF. Congenital nasal pyriform aperture stenosis. Arch Otolaryngol Head Neck Surg 1992;118:989–91.
3. Losken A, Burstein F, Williams J. Congenital nasal pyriform aperture stenosis: diagnosis and treatment. Plast Reconstr Surg 2002;109:1506–11.
4. Osovsky M, Aizer-Danon A, Horev G. Congenital pyriform aperture stenosis. Pediatr Radiol 2007;37:97–9.
5. Lee K, Yang C, Huang J, et al. Congenital pyriform aperture stenosis: surgery and evaluation with three dimensional computed tomography. Laryngoscope 2002; 112:918–21.
6. Levison J, Neas K, Wilson M, et al. Neonatal nasal obstruction and a single maxillary central incisor. J Paediatr Child Health 2005;41:380–1.
7. Van Den Abbeele T, Triglia JM, Francois M, et al. Congenital nasal pyriform stenosis: diagnosis and management of 20 cases. Ann Otol Rhinol Laryngol 2001;110:70–5.
8. Beregszazi M, Leger J, Garel C, et al. Nasal pyriform aperture stenosis and absence of the anterior pituitary gland: report of two cases. J Pediatr 1996;128: 858–61.
9. Vercruysse JP, Wojciechowski M, Koninckx M, et al. Congenital nasal pyriform aperture stenosis: a rare cause of neonatal nasal obstruction. J Pediatr Surg 2006;41:E5–7.
10. Lee J, Bent J, Ward R. Congenital nasal pyriform aperture stenosis: non-surgical management and long-term analysis. Int J Pediatr Otorhinolaryngol 2001;60: 167–72.
11. Hui Y, Friedber J, Crysdale WS. Congenital nasal pyriform aperture stenosis as a presenting feature of holoprosencephaly. Int J Pediatr Otorhinolaryngol 1995; 31:263–74.
12. Shikowitz M. Congenital nasal pyriform aperture stenosis: diagnosis and treatment [case report]. Int J Pediatr Otorhinolaryngol 2003;67:635–9.

Septoplasty Pearls

Eric J. Dobratz, MD[a,b], Stephen S. Park, MD[c,d],*

KEYWORDS

- Septoplasty • Deviated septum • Nasal septal deviation
- Nasal obstruction • Septal deformity • Nasal deformity
- Nasal valve obstruction • Extracorporeal septoplasty

The predominant surgical treatment for obstructive deviation of the nasal septum during the first half of the twentieth century was to perform a submucous resection (SMR). The SMR was initially popularized by Killian and Freer in the early 1900s to allow for removal of bony and cartilaginous deformities of the nasal septum. During SMR, deformities of the dorsal and caudal portions of the septum are not addressed in order to prevent postoperative saddle nose deformities and a retracted columella. Often, the septal deformities are removed, and straight pieces of cartilage or bone are not replaced.

In 1948, Cottle and Loring[1] published an article describing a new operative procedure on the nasal septum that allowed the surgeon to address deformities in all portions of the septum in addition to avoiding postoperative deformities. In that article, Cottle and Loring those researchers described the disadvantages of performing a Killian type incision near the mucocutaneous junction or more posterior. It is difficult to treat areas of obstruction located anterior to the Killian incision. They also described some disadvantages associated with bisecting the mucosal flaps, including the disruption of normal ciliary activity and interruption of the blood supply to the flap that feeds the replaced bone or cartilage.

Cottle and Loring[1] described the importance of addressing all portions of the bony and cartilaginous septum that are deviated. They stated that one should not hesitate to remove all the bone or cartilage that interferes with the normal passage of air in the nose. Once the airway is improved, they recommend replacing trimmed, thinned, and straightened pieces of septum between the mucosal flaps. Placing these pieces

a Department of Otolaryngology Head and Neck Surgery, University of Minnesota, 420 Delaware Street, MMC 396, Minneapolis, MN 55455, USA
b Facial Plastic and Reconstructive Surgery, University of Minnesota, 420 Delaware Street, MMC 396, Minneapolis, MN 55455, USA
c Department of Otolaryngology Head and Neck Surgery, University of Virginia, PO Box 800713, Charlottesville, VA 22908–0713, USA
d Division of Facial Plastic Surgery, University of Virginia, PO Box 800713, Charlottesville, VA 22908–0713, USA
* Corresponding author. Department of Otolaryngology Head and Neck Surgery, PO Box 800713, Charlottesville, VA 22908–0713.
E-mail address: ssp8a@virginia.edu (S.S. Park).

Otolaryngol Clin N Am 42 (2009) 527–537
doi:10.1016/j.otc.2009.03.003
0030-6665/09/$ – see front matter © 2009 Elsevier Inc. All rights reserved.

of cartilage provides support and, more importantly, prevents postoperative scar formation. This reduces contracture and subsequent deformity.

GENERAL APPROACH

The authors have found that caudal and dorsal septal deformities often contribute to the patient's obstruction. For this reason, they believe that a hemitransfixion incision and the approach described by Cottle and Loring[1] provide the best opportunity to treat deformities in these and other areas of the septum. They have also found it to be beneficial to preserve as much of the cartilaginous septum as possible and to replace excised portions with straightened septal grafts. They typically liberally excise bony irregularities, taking care to preserve the keystone area at the nasion.

The hemitransfixion incision and initial elevation of the mucoperichondrial flap are performed on the concave side of the cartilaginous septal deformity. The bony-cartilaginous junction is then separated, and mucoperiosteal flaps are raised bilaterally. The bony septum is then addressed. The authors attempt to treat the cartilaginous portion without raising the opposite mucosal flap. By elevating on the concave side, one can perform scoring maneuvers on the appropriate surface of the septal deformity. If scoring does not adequately treat the deformity, they move on to raise the contralateral flap and perform vertical slats or excision of portions of the cartilaginous septum. If the cartilaginous septum has a severe deformity or deviations in critical portions of the septum, they may perform explantation and reimplantation of the cartilage.

One of the most common cartilaginous septal deformities that the authors have encountered is that of an overly long quadrangular cartilage that is projected off of the maxillary crest in one side of the nasal cavity with subsequent bowing of the cartilage into the other side of the nose. This type of deformity can be treated by excising an inferior strip of the septum and placing the new inferior border on the maxillary crest.

Septal spurs, cartilaginous and bony, are also commonly encountered and are found to contribute to nasal obstruction. In this case, the authors often raise the mucosal flap on the side of the spur first. A tunnel is raised superior and inferior to the spur. The cartilaginous spur can then be separated from the septum and carefully freed from its lateral most attachments. Many times, the quadrangular cartilage and mucoperichondrial flap on the opposite side do not need to be violated. This provides the surgeon with the best opportunity to ensure that one of the flaps maintains its integrity and is not perforated. The bony or cartilaginous attachment can then be separated, and the bony septum can be addressed as usual.

In the upcoming sections, the authors describe some specific "pearls" that they have found helpful in treating patients with difficult-to-treat nasal septal deformities. They believe that the application of these pearls leads to increased satisfaction and decreased rates of revision surgery for patients.

Pearl 1: Don't Miss The Nasal Valve

The anatomy, dysfunction, and treatment of the nasal valve have been well described. A recent study points out that even among otolaryngologists, however, there continues to be "uncertainty and unease of sorts in defining the nasal valve component regions."[2] In a recent study, the authors found that 51% of patients undergoing revision septoplasty required treatment of the nasal valve to correct their nasal airway obstruction.[3] In contrast, only 4% of patients who underwent treatment of the valve during a primary septoplasty required revision surgery for nasal obstruction. They surmise that there are two main explanations for these data: (1) the surgeon is missing the contribution of the nasal valve before the primary surgery or (2) the patient develops narrowing of the valve over time.

In some instances, it is likely that both are contributing causes of the patient's continued airway obstruction. Therefore, it is important assess the anatomy of the nasal valve to determine if there is dysfunction at the valve.

The internal nasal valve is bounded by the nasal septum, the caudal border of the upper lateral cartilage, and the lateral nasal wall at the level of the anterior surface of the inferior turbinate. Dysfunction of the internal valve may be attributable to collapse of the upper lateral cartilage toward the septum, dorsal deviation of the septum toward the valve, or a combination of both. Collapse of the caudal border of the upper lateral cartilage may be dynamic, static, or both. Determining the cause of the internal valve obstruction is necessary to determine the correct approach for treatment.

Static obstruction of the internal nasal valve attributable to collapsed upper lateral cartilage may be treated by placement of a spreader graft or flaring suture.[4] In this study, the combination of flaring sutures and spreader grafts provided the greatest impact on the cross-sectional area of the nasal valve (**Fig. 1**). Some patients have static obstruction attributable to a dorsal septal deviation at the location of the valve with or without collapse of the upper lateral cartilage as well. In these instances, the dorsal deflection must be addressed in addition to the upper lateral cartilage. This is described in further detail in the next section (pearl 2). These patients are often treated with a spreader graft to splint the dorsal septum and treat the valve. A flaring suture may be incorporated as well.

Dynamic collapse of the nasal sidewall can contribute to nasal obstruction as well. Dorsal or caudal deflections of the septum can often accentuate the obstruction caused by collapse of the sidewall. In these instances, one should treat the septal deflection in addition to the sidewall collapse. Collapse of the nasal sidewall or vestibule may be attributable to deformity in the area of the external valve or intervalve. The external valve deformity is rare, and treatment is directed at relieving the cause of cicatricial stenosis causing the deformity. The authors have found that dynamic valve

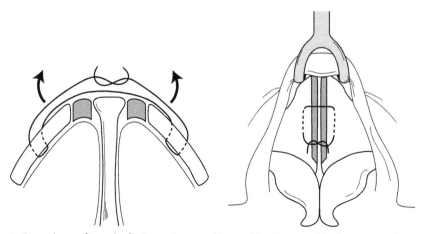

Fig. 1. Spreader grafts and a flaring suture used in combination provide the greatest increase in cross-sectional area of the internal valve. This is used for static collapse of the internal nasal valve.

obstruction is most frequently attributable to dysfunction at the intervalve area. The intervalve area is located at the caudal edge of the lateral crus, extending laterally toward the piriform aperture, including the area of the sesamoid cartilages. Collapse in this area often corresponds to a deep supra-alar crease and is treated by the placement of septal or auricular cartilage batten grafts. It is imperative that these grafts extend laterally over the piriform aperture to provide adequate support. In cases in which there is paradoxical concavity of the lateral crura, a lateral crural flip-flop graft may be performed. Lateral crural strut grafts or batten grafts may be used for recurvature of the lower lateral cartilage.

Spreader and batten grafts can be placed through endonasal and external approaches. The authors have found it best to place these grafts through an external approach. They believe this allows for better visualization in addition to precise and secure placement of the grafts. The external approach also allows the surgeon to place a flaring suture to improve the cross-sectional area of the internal valve further.

Pearl 2: Don't Miss The Dorsal Deviation

When evaluating a patient with septal deviation, one's attention is often drawn to deviations in the posterior or bony septum and to septal spurs. Caudal septal deformities are generally easy to diagnose yet more difficult to treat because of the importance of the support provided by the caudal portion of the septum. The authors have found, however, that deviations of the dorsal portion of the septum are often missed and frequently contribute significantly to the symptoms of nasal obstruction. It is difficult to know if dorsal deviations are noted but not treated because of the difficulty in accessing this area through traditional endonasal septoplasty approaches. Alternatively, deviations in this area may go unrecognized during the initial evaluation and treatment. Significant dorsal deviations of the septum can also result in significant deviations of the external appearance of the nose, resulting in a crooked nose deformity. As stated previously, dorsal deflections in the area of the caudal portion of the upper lateral cartilage accentuate nasal obstruction by contributing to internal nasal valve obstruction.

Although others have described treating dorsal irregularities through an endonasal or endoscopic approach, the authors have found it best to treat significant dorsal deformities through an external rhinoplasty approach. This allows the surgeon the opportunity to disarticulate the attachments of the mucoperichondrium and upper lateral cartilages to the dorsal portion of the septum and provides for complete and unobstructed access to the dorsal septum. It is also important to note that dorsal septal irregularities are not addressed through the SMR technique.

A chart summarizing the treatment of dorsal septal deviations causing nasal obstruction is shown in **Fig. 2**. It is important first to free all the attachments from the dorsal septum. Freeing the dorsal septum occasionally allows the dorsal septum to straighten out, permitting the surgeon to reattach the upper lateral cartilages, resulting in adequate improvement of the airway and more a straightened appearance of the nasal dorsum. Often, the intrinsic deformity of the cartilage requires other maneuvers to straighten the septum appropriately. The concave portion of the deflection may be scored to release some of the intrinsic deformity that exists in the cartilage. In more severe cases, vertical slats may be placed into the dorsal strut; however, these should not extend up within 5 mm of the dorsal edge of the strut (**Fig. 3**). If vertical slats are made into the dorsal strut, or if there is continued deformity, unilateral or bilateral spreader grafts should be placed to provide support and to act as a splint to straighten the dorsal deviation.

Some patients present with unilateral collapse of the upper lateral cartilage and dorsal deflection of the septum, resulting in internal nasal valve dysfunction. The

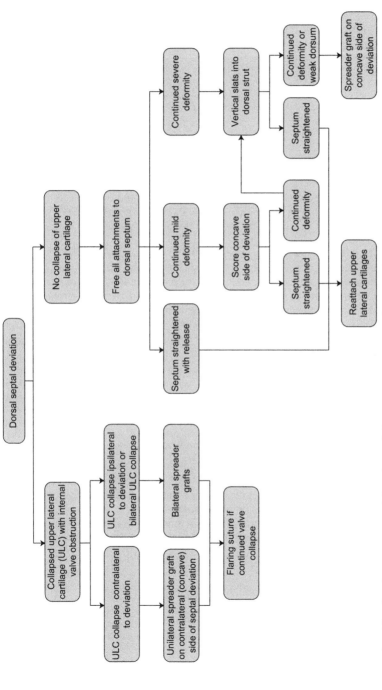

Fig. 2. An algorithm for the treatment of dorsal septal deviations causing nasal airway obstruction.

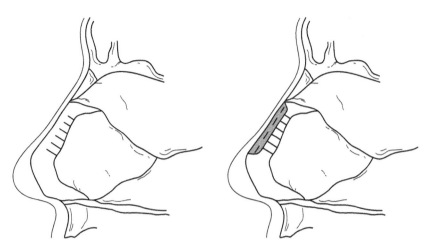

Fig. 3. (*Left*) Vertical slats placed into the dorsal strut. (*Right*) If there is continued deformity or weakening of the dorsal strut, unilateral or bilateral spreader grafts should be placed to provide support and to act as a splint to straighten the dorsal deviation.

collapsed upper lateral cartilage may be ipsilateral to the concave side of the dorsal deflection. These patients often also have the appearance of a crooked nose because of a dorsal septal deviation that is accentuated by a middle vault depression on the opposite side. These patients benefit from placement of a unilateral spreader graft on the concave side of the deflection. The graft helps to splint the dorsal septum and opens up the nasal valve by providing support for and lateralizing the upper lateral cartilage. This results in an improved and more symmetric appearance of the nasal dorsum in the middle vault on that side as well.

Other patients have valve obstruction on the convex side of the dorsal deflection. These patients require bilateral spreader grafts, with one graft on the concave side to splint the septum. The other graft is used to lateralize the depressed upper lateral cartilage.

Pearl 3: Complex Deformities May Require Explantation

Patients who have experienced repeated nasal trauma and those with a history of cleft lip or palate malformation may develop severe deformity of the septum. These patients often have deformities in critical support areas of the nasal septum that cannot be treated by resection, scoring, or incision techniques.

In 2005, Gubisch[5] described his experience of performing extracorporeal septoplasty on 2119 patients with severe septal deformity. In that study, he describes explanting the severely deformed septum and straightening the septum by various techniques. These techniques include the following:

- Excise and suture together redundant cartilage and fractures.
- Score areas of deformity.
- Drill down thick deformed portions of the septum.
- Suture areas of straight bony septum to areas of weak cartilaginous septum.
- Place spreader grafts for dorsal irregularity.
- Use polydioxanone foil as a template for stabilizing cartilage pieces.

He secures the reimplanted septum to the nasal spine and superiorly to the upper lateral cartilages or through transcutaneous suture through the nasal dorsum. This procedure has been successful; however, the most common complication encountered was development of dorsal irregularities. Saddling occurred more frequently during his early experience. The incidence of saddling decreased after he started securing the septum to the upper lateral cartilage.

Most[6] describes a modification of the extracorporeal septoplasty technique to decrease the incidence of developing dorsal irregularities. He advocates the following:

- Resecting only the anterior cartilaginous septum
- Avoiding destabilization of the keystone area
- Preserving the dorsal contour

He describes this procedure as an anterior septal reconstruction (ASR). He resects most of the cartilaginous septum, although leaving a 1.5-cm dorsal strut. An open rhinoplasty is performed, and the straightened ASR graft is then secured to the concave side of the dorsal septum remnant, which acts as a spreader graft and septal splint.

The authors perform variations of the extracorporeal septoplasty described by Gubisch[5] and the ASR described by Most[6] depending on the degree and location of the deviation encountered. For patients with a minimal deformity of the dorsal septum but with severe deviation in other portions of cartilaginous septum, they leave a dorsal strut and resect the remainder of the cartilaginous septum. This is performed through an endonasal approach, and the upper lateral cartilages remain attached to the dorsal septum. The dorsal septum remains attached to the bony septum as well, allowing maintenance of the dorsal profile. A straight portion of the resected cartilage that is at least 1.5 cm wide is then fashioned as a caudal strut (**Fig. 4**). The cartilage is placed over the remaining maxillary crest, and the inferior portion is secured to the periosteum of the maxillary spine using 5-0 clear nylon suture. The superior portion is then sutured to the remaining dorsal cartilaginous strut.

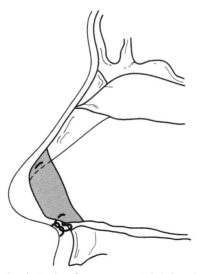

Fig. 4. Explantation and reimplantation for severe septal deformities with a straight dorsal septum. A straight caudal strut is secured to the native dorsal strut, which is left intact, and also to the periosteum of the nasal spine.

In patients with a significant cartilaginous deformity that includes the dorsum, the entire cartilaginous septum is excised except for a small portion that is left intact with the bony dorsal septum located beneath the nasion. This small portion of cartilage is just large enough to provide support and an area for reattachment of an L-shaped septal strut graft. Once the L-shaped septal strut is created, it is sutured to the remnant of the dorsal caudal septum that is attached to the bony septum (**Fig. 5**). As stated previously, when addressing significant dorsal irregularities, the authors have found it best to perform an external approach. Thus, they have not found it necessary to perform transcutaneous sutures to provide support. The upper lateral cartilages are then secured to the new straightened dorsum. The base of the caudal strut is then secured to the maxillary spine to stabilize the graft.

Pearl 4: Septal Suturing—No Packing Needed

Otolaryngologists typically place packing or quilting sutures on the completion of the septoplasty to coapt the mucosal flaps, avoid septal hematoma, and provide support. Nasal packing creates a significant amount of discomfort for patients. Alternatives to packing have been sought, and successful coaptation of the flaps by means of septal suturing has been described.[7,8] In a recent prospective study, patients undergoing septal suturing versus nasal packing were compared. Patients who underwent suturing had similar outcomes and less discomfort than patients undergoing nasal packing.[9]

The authors perform a quilting suture using a 4-0 chromic gut suture as follows:

- The suture is passed through and through the nasal septum as far posterior as possible along the floor of the nose.
- The suture is then passed anteriorly and superiorly back towards the columella.
- A series of interrupted chromic sutures is then passed through the caudal and membranous septum, recreating support in the area of the hemitransfixion incision. These sutures also close the incision.

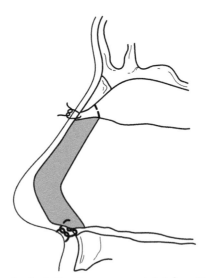

Fig. 5. Explantation and reimplantation for severe septal deformities with significant deviation in the dorsal septum. A straight L-shaped strut is secured to a small portion of cartilage that is left attached to the bony septum at the keystone area. The inferior portion of the caudal end of the graft is secured to the periosteum of the nasal spine.

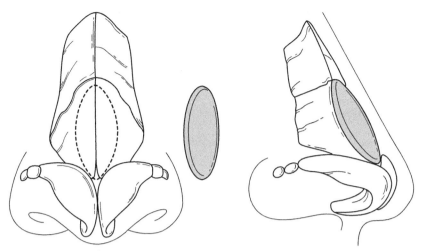

Fig. 6. For patients with a subtle depression and stable midvault, a small canoe-shaped cartilage graft is placed in a small tunnel that is created over the middle of the dorsum. The tunnel is created through an intercartilaginous incision.

Table 1
Summary of five pearls that can increase patient satisfaction after septoplasty for nasal airway obstruction

Pearl	Description
Don't miss the nasal valve	51% of patients undergoing revision septoplasty required treatment of the nasal valve to correct their nasal airway obstruction
Don't miss the dorsal deviation	The authors have found it best to treat significant dorsal deformities through an external rhinoplasty approach. Dorsal deviations are not addressed through the SMR technique.
Complex deformities may require explantation	Patients with severe deformity of the septum often have deviations in critical support areas that cannot be treated by resection, scoring, or incision techniques. These patients require explantation with reimplantation of a straightened portion of the septum for support.
Septal suturing—no packing needed	Studies have shown that patients who underwent septal suturing had similar outcomes and less discomfort than patients undergoing nasal packing.
Dorsal onlay to correct subtle "saddling"	When the middle vault support feels adequate but a small depression is noted on profile view, the authors have found it beneficial to place a dorsal onlay graft for camouflaging the depression.

- Finally, one suture is placed under the domes at the anterior septal angle and then through the membranous septum, helping to support the nasal tip.

They believe that this suturing technique provides adequate approximation of the flaps with minimal discomfort. It also provides the opportunity to place key support sutures along the caudal border of the septum, however, recreating some of the support that is disrupted during the hemitransfixion incision while the area is healing and scarring in place.

Pearl 5: Dorsal Onlay To Correct Subtle "Saddling"

The upper lateral cartilaginous vault consists of the paired upper lateral cartilages and their fusion with the dorsal septum from the nasal bones to the septal angle. In performing various maneuvers to address septal deviation, there is an increased risk for developing instability of the septum, leading to the development of a saddle nose deformity. Patients with congenitally small, short, or thin upper lateral cartilages and injured upper lateral cartilages are at greater risk for a sagging cartilaginous dorsum after surgery because of weakening of the midline and lateral supports of the middle vault. At the conclusion of the treatment of septal deformities, the middle vault in all patients should be assessed and palpated. If there are signs of weakening, it is important to place dorsal or septal grafts to support this area.

When the middle vault support feels adequate but a small depression is noted on profile view, the authors have found it beneficial to place a dorsal onlay graft for camouflaging the depression. A small piece of septal cartilage is carved into a canoe shape. This is placed through an intercartilaginous incision. A small tunnel is created over the middle of the dorsum, and the graft is placed to fill in the depression (**Fig. 6**). Care is taken to create the tunnel so that there is not excess room for the graft to move in. The edges of the graft are beveled to ensure that the edges are not palpable.

SUMMARY

The difficulty of treating septal deformities that lead to nasal airway obstruction varies significantly depending on the location and severity of the deformity. In this article, the authors have provided surgeons with a set of technical and diagnostic pearls to assist them in treating patients with nasal septal deformities causing nasal obstruction (**Table 1**). The techniques that the authors have described should assist the surgeon in treating patients with difficult-to-treat nasal septal deformities, including dorsal deflections of the septum and severe septal deformities. It is imperative for surgeons to analyze the nasal valve while evaluating septal deformities, because a dysfunctional nasal valve frequently contributes to the patient's symptoms airway obstruction. The placement of quilting sutures without nasal packing allows for equivalent flap coaptation without the significant discomfort of the nasal pack. The specific placement of key sutures also helps to provide support as the tissues are healing and scar into place. Finally, patients with subtle saddling and adequate support may benefit from the placement of a small dorsal onlay graft to camouflage the depression. The authors believe that the application of the pearls they have described leads to increased satisfaction and decreased rates of revision surgery for patients.

REFERENCES

1. Cottle MH, Loring RM. Surgery of the nasal septum—new operative procedures and indications. Ann Otol Rhinol Laryngol 1948;57:705–13.

2. Wexler DB, Davidson TM. The nasal valve: a review of the anatomy, imaging, and physiology. Am J Rhinol 2004;18:143–50.
3. Becker SS, Dobratz EJ, Stowell N, et al. Revision septoplasty: review of sources of persistent nasal obstruction. Am J Rhinol 2008;22:440–4.
4. Schlosser RJ, Park SS. Surgery for the dysfunctional nasal valve. Cadaveric analysis and clinical outcomes. Arch Facial Plast Surg 1999;1:105–10.
5. Gubisch W. Extracorporeal septoplasty for the markedly deviated septum. Arch Facial Plast Surg 2005;7:218–26.
6. Most SP. Anterior septal reconstruction: outcomes after a modified extracorporeal septoplasty technique. Arch Facial Plast Surg 2006;8:202–7.
7. Sessions RB. Membrane approximation by continuous mattress sutures following septoplasty. Laryngoscope 1984;94(Pt 1):702–3.
8. Lee IN, Vukovic L. Hemostatic suture for septoplasty: how we do it. J Otolaryngol 1988;17:54–6.
9. Al-Raggad DK, El-Jundi AM, Al-Momani OS, et al. Suturing of the nasal septum after septoplasty, is it an effective alternative to nasal packing? Saudi Med J 2007;28(10):1534–6.

Cosmetic and Functional Effects of Cephalic Malposition of the Lower Lateral Cartilages: A Facial Plastic Surgical Case Study

Cory C. Yeh, MD[a,b,*], Edwin F. Williams III, MD[a,b]

KEYWORDS

- Rhinoplasty • Cephalic malposition • External nasal valve
- Alar cartilage • Lower lateral cartilage

L.B. is a 35-year-old female who presented with nasal obstruction and a nasal deformity. She had a history of trauma to her nose when she was accidentally struck by a golf club at the age of 15. She had an attempted closed reduction of the nasal fracture at that time and now complains of persistent left- and right-side nasal obstruction. Additionally, she was concerned about the appearance of her nose and disliked the large size and fullness of the tip. A review of systems and her past medical history was unremarkable. Physical examination with attention to nasal analysis revealed a nose with an acute nasolabial angle that is overprojected. Analysis of the nasal septum revealed a C-shaped deformity to the left. The nasal tip appeared to have a boxy configuration with significantly medially rotated supra-alar creases. A hanging columella was identified. The external valves were deficient bilaterally with incomplete collapse on inspiration (**Fig. 1**).

The patient underwent a rhinoplasty using an endonasal approach. A septoplasty was performed first to correct the C-shaped deformity. Cephalic malposition of the lower lateral cartilages, which was suspected preoperatively, was confirmed

[a] Williams Center Plastic Surgery Specialists, 1072 Troy-Schenectady Road, Latham, NY 12110, USA
[b] Facial Plastic and Reconstructive Surgery, Division of Otolaryngology-Head and Neck Surgery, Department of Surgery, Albany Medical Center, Albany, NY, USA
* Corresponding author. Williams Center Plastic Surgery Specialists, 1072 Troy-Schenectady Road, Latham, NY 12110.
E-mail address: coryyeh@gmail.com (C.C. Yeh).

Otolaryngol Clin N Am 42 (2009) 539–546
doi:10.1016/j.otc.2009.03.007
0030-6665/09/$ – see front matter © 2009 Elsevier Inc. All rights reserved.

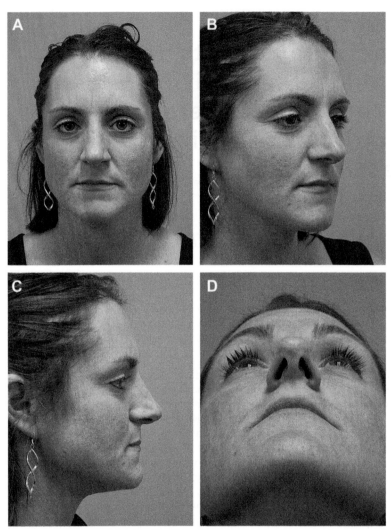

Fig. 1. Patient L.B. preoperative photos. (*A*) Anterior view. (*B*) Oblique view. (*C*) Profile view. (*D*) Base view.

intraoperatively. A conservative cephalic trim was performed through an intracartilaginous incision with careful attention paid to identifying the true cephalic border of the alar cartilage. Cartilage harvested from the cephalic trim was weakened and placed as an alar rim graft bilaterally through a small pocket created along the mid ala. A tongue-in-groove suture was placed to reduce the hanging columella, and medial and lateral osteotomies were performed to correct the position of the nasal bones (**Fig. 2**).

Postoperatively, the patient was pleased with her rhinoplasty results, particularly the correction of her tip deformity. Her nasal breathing was improved and there was no further evidence of external nasal valve collapse on inspiration (**Fig. 3**).

Rhinoplasty is a surgical procedure that requires a meticulous nasal evaluation, while simultaneously challenging the surgeon's judgment and technical execution.

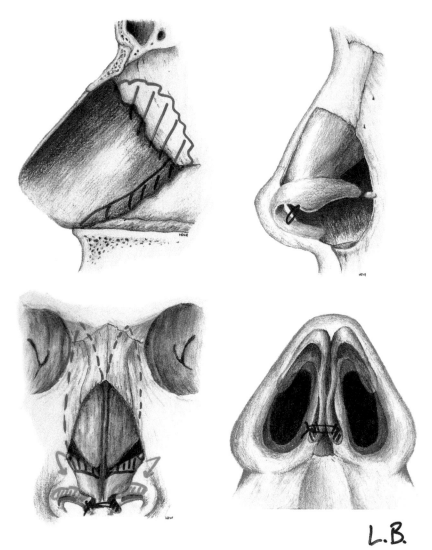

Fig. 2. Patient L.B. operative rhinoplasty worksheet. Operative maneuvers include resection of septal cartilage and bone (*red hash marks*), medial and lateral osteotomies (*red dotted lines*), tongue-in-groove septal-crural suture (*blue loop*), and cephalic trim of the lower lateral cartilage (*red hash marks*) with replacement as a free graft along the alar rim (*green hash marks*).

The time spent critically analyzing the patient's nasal anatomy allows the surgeon to appreciate the individual contributions of the underlying bone, cartilage framework, and skin and soft tissue envelope to the nasal shape and form. This evaluation should include both careful inspection of the nasal topography and thorough palpation of the cartilage framework and skin. Surgeons who fail to recognize functional nasal abnormalities or inadvertently create breathing problems from a rhinoplasty are not maximizing their patients' outcomes.

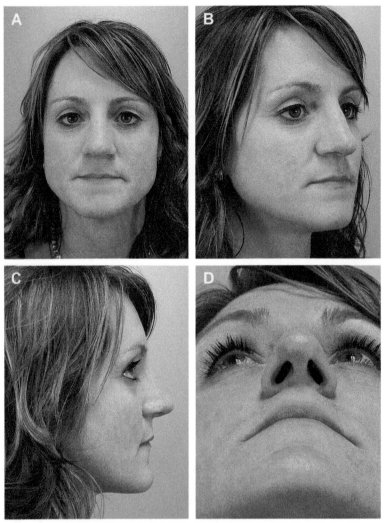

Fig. 3. Patient L.B. 2.5-months postoperative photos. (*A*) Anterior view. (*B*) Oblique view. (*C*) Profile view. (*D*) Base view.

CEPHALIC MALPOSITION: COMMON ANATOMIC VARIATION

Cephalic malposition of the paired lower lateral cartilages is a common anatomic variation of the underlying cartilage framework. Normally, the lateral crura follow the curvature of the alar margin before diverging at a 30 to 45° angle toward the lateral canthus at the mid ala. Sheen[1] was one of the first to describe the cephalic malposition abnormality, in which the lateral crura diverge early and at a greater than 45° angle from the alar margin toward the ipsilateral medial canthus. This anatomic variation occurs commonly as illustrated in multiple reports by Constantian.[2–5] In his study of 200 consecutive primary and secondary rhinoplasty patients, the majority of the patients had alar cartilage malposition. Sixty-eight percent of primary rhinoplasty patients and 87% of secondary rhinoplasty patients manifested this anatomic abnormality.[5] In an earlier study, Constantian found that cephalic malposition of the alar cartilage occurred at lower rates with 18% of primary rhinoplasty patients and up to 42% of secondary rhinoplasty patients affected. While this may be a reflection of selection bias to a specific rhinoplasty practice, it is more important to realize that this anatomic abnormality was found to strongly predispose a patient to unfavorable rhinoplasty results.[4] It is clear that the effect of cephalic malposition of the lower lateral cartilages on both the cosmetic nasal contour and functional nasal breathing is frequently underappreciated.

CEPHALIC MALPOSITION: COSMETIC DEFORMITY

Cephalic malposition of the alar cartilages can result in a significant cosmetic nasal deformity. Classically, this has been referred to as a "parenthesis tip deformity" where the supra-alar crease is moved medially and cephalically oriented, thereby resembling a pair of parenthesis that frames the nasal tip. Additionally, it has also been recognized that varying degrees of cephalic malposition can create characteristic configurations of the nasal tip. Constantian[5] was the first to emphasize that "boxy" and "ball" nasal tips, long recognized as common configurations of the lower third of the nose, may in fact be directly associated with the cephalic malposition abnormality. In his study of 200 consecutive primary and secondary rhinoplasty patients, most of the primary (74%) and secondary patients (76%) with alar cartilage malposition had either boxy or ball nasal tips. In this study, Constantian also found that patients who present with a boxy or ball nasal tip have seven times the likelihood of having malpositioned, rather than orthotopic lower lateral crura.

CEPHALIC MALPOSITION: AIRFLOW OBSTRUCTION

Cephalic malposition of the alar cartilages can also result in a significant obstruction to nasal airflow. The obstruction is usually due to a deficiency of support at the external nasal valve. This valve, which is framed by the nostril sill inferiorly, alar rim circumferentially, and inferior turbinate posteriorly, is dependent upon the alar cartilage shape and structure for maintaining an open anterior nasal airway. With cephalic malposition, the majority of the alar cartilage is directly cephalically toward the ipsilateral medial canthus and therefore away from the mid alar margin and lateral ala. This divergence results in weakness of the external valve, particularly along its lateral border. These patients will commonly complain of a reduction in nasal airflow on the affected side. In cases of severe external nasal valve weakness, the lateral ala can completely collapse on inspiration resulting in severe nasal obstruction. In a report of 61 patients with external nasal valve collapse, 27 of those patients (47%) had alar cartilage malposition.[3]

RHINOPLASTY ANATOMIC ANALYSIS

Most investigators agree that the most critical step in a rhinoplasty procedure is a thorough preoperative anatomic nasal evaluation. Weakness of the external or internal nasal valves can be readily appreciated through simple physical examination maneuvers. At this time, an analysis of the surface topography of the nose can reveal the presence or absence of cephalic malposition of the alar cartilages. As described above, one should be suspicious of a cephalically positioned lower lateral cartilage in a patient who presents with a boxy or ball nasal tip. Further, patients with a medially rotated and vertically positioned supra-alar crease have a high likelihood for underlying cephalic malposition. Although it may be difficult, particularly for the novice surgeon, to make this anatomic diagnosis with certainty preoperatively, it is more important that he or she be prepared at the time of surgery to modify the techniques to avoid iatrogenic injury to the malpositioned cartilage.

OPEN RHINOPLASTY APPROACH

In an open rhinoplasty approach, elevation of the skin and soft tissue envelope will readily reveal the presence of cephalically rotated alar cartilages. If the patient has external nasal valve collapse or desires correction of a tip deformity that is secondary to cephalic malposition, there are multiple options for surgical correction. These include repair of the external nasal valve through either a batten graft or placement of an alar rim graft in patients with a weak alar margin. Often, the cartilage graft material for the batten or alar rim graft can be obtained through a judicious cephalic trim of the lower lateral cartilage, which should be performed first. Other options for cartilage grafting include septal or conchal cartilage. If the patient desires a cosmetic rhinoplasty with alteration of the nasal tip, the surgeon may need to use cartilage-repositioning techniques.[6] In these cases, the cephalic lower lateral cartilage is rotated laterally and inferiorly and sutured into position adjacent to the sesamoid cartilages. Without placement of alar batten grafts or cartilage repositioning techniques, there is significant risk of cephalic alar retraction in the open rhinoplasty approach. This phenomenon is secondary to scar contracture forces between the alar margin and the cephalic malpositioned alar cartilage through susceptible intervening soft tissue.[7]

ENDONASAL RHINOPLASTY APPROACH

Surgeons who prefer an endonasal rhinoplasty approach commonly cite less postoperative edema, quicker healing, and a more reliable immediate feedback of changes in nasal contour intraoperatively as distinct advantages from the open approach. If one fails to recognize alar cartilage malposition and performs a cephalic trim of the lower

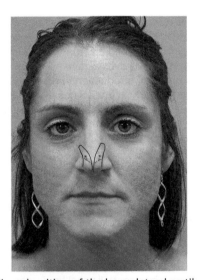

Fig. 4. Patient L.B. cephalic malposition of the lower lateral cartilages. A standard intracartilaginous incision using an endonasal rhinoplasty approach would inadvertently transect the cartilage along the dotted line.

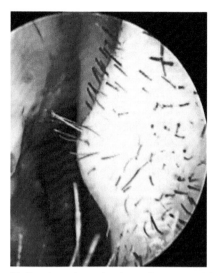

Fig. 5. Endoscopic view of left external nasal valve collapse secondary to cephalic malposition of the lower lateral cartilages.

lateral cartilage through a standard intracartilaginous incision, the cephalically positioned alar cartilage is at risk for complete transection (**Figs. 4** and **5**). This may actually exacerbate the underlying airway problem by further weakening the external nasal valve. Therefore, it is critical to identify this abnormality to avoid severe iatrogenic injury to the cartilage framework. Cartilage repositioning techniques can be performed endonasally in experienced hands, but this has a somewhat steeper learning curve than the open rhinoplasty approach. In some patients, it may be easier to strengthen the external nasal valve with a batten graft or alar rim graft obtained as a free graft from a correctly positioned cephalic trim resection. These grafts are typically placed by positioning the cartilage graft into a soft tissue pocket created through a marginal incision. The use of cartilage grafts to strengthen the external nasal valve can result in dramatic improvement of the underlying nasal obstruction. In one study, rhinomanometry measurements after correction of an external nasal valve collapse secondary to cephalic malposition by way of an endonasal approach showed doubling of the geometric mean nasal airflow.[3]

SUMMARY: CEPHALIC MALPOSITION

In summary, cephalic malposition of the lower lateral cartilages is a frequent anatomic variation of nasal anatomy. Alar cartilage malposition results in cosmetic changes to nasal contour including nasal tip fullness and characteristic tip configurations such as the boxy tip, ball tip, or parentheses tip. Further, cephalic malposition is often associated with significant external nasal valve weakness that can result in nasal obstruction. The surgeon must become facile with an analysis of surface topography to suspect alar cartilage malposition preoperatively to avoid iatrogenic injury to the lower lateral cartilage during standard rhinoplasty maneuvers. If external valve collapse is present, an open approach or endonasal approach can be used to strengthen the valve through placement of batten or alar rim grafts, or through cartilage repositioning techniques.

REFERENCES

1. Sheen JH. Aesthetic rhinoplasty. St. Louis (MO): Mosby; 1978. p. 432–62.
2. Constantian MB. The incompetent external nasal valve: pathophysiology and treatment in primary and secondary rhinoplasty. Plast Reconstr Surg 1994;93(5): 919–31.
3. Constantian MB. Functional effects of alar cartilage malposition. Ann Plast Surg 1993;30(6):487–99.
4. Constantian MB. Four common anatomic variants that predispose to unfavorable rhinoplasty results: a study based on 150 consecutive secondary rhinoplasties. Plast Reconstr Surg 2000;105(1):316–31.
5. Constantian MB. The boxy nasal tip, the ball tip, and alar cartilage malposition: variations on a theme—a study in 200 consecutive primary and secondary rhinoplasty patients. Plast Reconstr Surg 2005;116(1):268–81.
6. Hamra ST. Repositioning the lateral alar crus. Plast Reconstr Surg 1993;92(7): 1244–53.
7. Shah AR, Miller PJ. Structural approach to endonasal rhinoplasty. Facial Plast Surg 2006;22(1):55–60.

Nasal Reconstruction of the Leprosy Nose Using Costal Cartilage

Anil R. Shah, MD[a,b], Daniel Zeitler, MD[a], Jeffrey B. Wise, MD[c,d],*

KEYWORDS

- Saddle-nose deformity • Leprosy
- Autogenous costal cartilage graft • Rhinoplasty
- Nasal reconstruction

Leprosy is a chronic granulomatous infection of the soft tissue of the skin and peripheral nerves that has plagued industrialized human populations worldwide for thousands of years. Leprosy remains a commonly occurring disease in some countries, with over 219,000 cases reported and a prevalence of more than one case per 10,000 people.[1] Unfortunately, despite medications that can effectively treat leprosy, it remains a difficult disease to detect, and diagnosis often occurs after the onset of several specific deformities. One of the most common manifestations of leprosy is the destruction of nasal cartilage. Interestingly, this disease universally preserves the skin, mucosa, and lower lateral cartilages of the nose.

Believed to have originated in the Indian subcontinent, the disease traversed the globe from Europe to Africa, along with the Far East and South America. However, since the description of the causative etiologic agent, *Mycobacterium leprae*, in 1873 by Gerhard HA Hansen, the disease has become concentrated mostly in resource-poor countries within tropical climate zones. Currently, 83% of recorded cases of the disease are found in only six countries: India, Brazil, Burma, Indonesia, Madagascar, and Nepal.[2] Because of the large immigrant influx into major metropolitan cities within the United States, coupled with leprosy patients frequently presenting with signs and symptoms of the disease long after leaving an endemic region, it is important that clinicians in the United States be able to diagnose and treat manifestations of this disease.

[a] Division of Facial Plastic Surgery, Section of Otolaryngology, University of Chicago, 845 North Michican Avenue, Suite 934e, Chicago, IL 60611, USA
[b] Private Practice, 845 North Michican Avenue, Suite 934e, Chicago, IL 60611, USA
[c] Division of Facial Plastic Surgery, Department of Otolaryngology, New York University School of Medicine, New York, NY, USA
[d] Private Practice, 1680 Route 23, Suite 100, Wayne, NJ 07470, USA
* Corresponding author. Division of Facial Plastic Surgery, Department of Otolaryngology, New York University School of Medicine, New York, NY.
E-mail address: jeffreywisemd@gmail.com (J.B. Wise).

Otolaryngol Clin N Am 42 (2009) 547–555
doi:10.1016/j.otc.2009.03.009
0030-6665/09/$ – see front matter © 2009 Elsevier Inc. All rights reserved.

Although there are numerous functional and cosmetic consequences secondary to lepromatous disease, perhaps none is more distressing or socially stigmatized than the development of a saddle-nose deformity. Inhalation of the mycobacterium allows for infiltration of the nasal mucosa and subsequent destruction of the bony and cartilaginous skeleton along with the mucosal lining.[3] This process results in extensive remodeling of the nasal framework and significant ensuing deformities. Surgeons have proposed a variety of reconstructive techniques, which include nasolabial turnover flaps,[4] post-nasal skin grafts,[5] silicone rubber implants and other external prostheses,[5] and most recently, autologous auricular and/or costal cartilage grafts.[6] This article presents a case of severe saddle-nose deformity secondary to prior infection with *Mycobacterium leprae* (leprosy), and successful reconstruction with autologous costal cartilage grafts.

CASE REPORT

A 37-year old female born in the Dominican Republic, and a recent immigrant to the United States, presented with a complaint of complete nasal collapse. Her pertinent history began 7 years previously at age 30, when she sought medical attention from a dermatologist for multiple skin lesions developing on her upper extremities and trunk. A diagnosis of leprosy was made based on histologic evidence, and the patient was treated for several months with "multiple antibiotics." Beginning in her mid-30s, the patient began to note progressive changes in the structure of her nose, along with significant nasal obstruction. Gradually, she noticed her entire nose "collapse." Family members and friends had difficulty recognizing her. The patient does not report a history of other family members contracting or having been treated for leprosy in the past. The leprosy has been "quiescent" for a period of 2 years since her last treatments, the details of which she did not recall.

Physical examination demonstrated a woman with a severe saddle nose deformity and total nasal septal perforation. The patient had decreased tip support and recoil, which resulted in a bulbous, underprojected nasal tip. Aside from significant middle vault collapse, she also demonstrated deficient premaxillary projection (**Fig. 1**).

A nasal reconstruction was performed via an open rhinoplasty approach. Costal cartilage from two ribs—specifically the left seventh and eighth ribs—were harvested to repair her nose. Support of the nasal base was achieved with an extended columellar strut, carved from costal cartilage. The strut was carved to help project the nasal tip and augment the columella and premaxilla. The strut was not integrated with the residual septum (**Fig. 2**) Two interrupted permanent sutures were placed through the periosteum along the nasal spine to stabilize the graft (**Figs. 3 and 4**). In an effort to augment the premaxilla, several small pieces of costal cartilage (2 mm × 2 mm × 2 mm) were placed in a precisely made intranasal pocket and closed with 4-0 chromic gut sutures (Ethicon, Somerville, New Jersey).

A mild boney dorsal reduction was undertaken with a rasping technique to allow for a smooth platform for nasal dorsum augmentation. A thinly-sculpted dorsal onlay graft was placed over the nasal bones and upper lateral cartilages. The graft was carved from the soft central core of costal cartilage in an effort to mitigate the risk of cartilaginous warping. Furthermore, a moderately-crushed cartilagenous graft was placed over the middle third. Finally, the radix was augmented with remaining costal perichondrium (see **Fig. 4**).

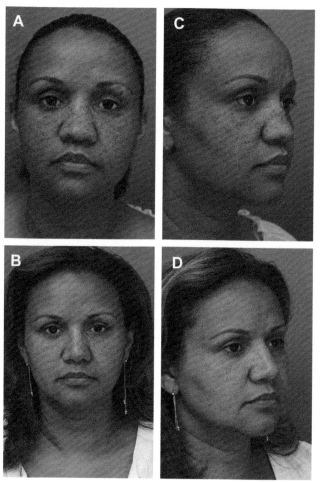

Fig. 1. Preoperative views in the frontal (*A*), lateral (*C*), oblique (*E*), and base respectively (*G*), demonstrating a severe saddle nose deformity. Note the relative absence of tip support, resulting in tip underprojection and bulbosity. On lateral view, deficient premaxillary projection is noted. Postoperative views at 1 year in the Frontal (*B*), Lateral (*D*), Oblique (*F*), and Base (*H*) respectively. There is significant improvement in dorsal height and in projection of the nasal tip and premaxilla. Nasal length has been augmented, and refinement of the nasal tip has been achieved.

LEPROSY EPIDEMIOLOGY

The pathology of nasal skeleton collapse in leprosy begins with nasal septal mucosal edema and subsequent destruction following infiltration with *Mycobacterium leprae*, an inhaled pathogen. The majority of patients with nasal collapse have long-standing disease.[3] Initially, the damage is microscopic; however, as the disease progresses, the destruction becomes visible on gross examination.[7] After the nasal septal mucosa is destroyed, the underlying quadrangular cartilage is exposed leading to secondary bacterial infection. Alternatively, exposure necrosis may result secondary to vascular ischemia, with the loss of the perichondrial blood supply. The end result is septal perforation. Those structures covered by respiratory mucosa on both surfaces,

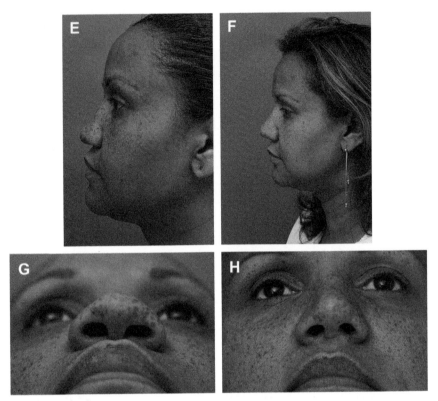

Fig. 1. (*continued*)

including the nasal septum, nasal spine of the maxilla, and the turbinates, are most prone to destruction. As the nasal spine is resorbed, the classic saddle-nose deformity can develop, accompanied by an acute nasolabial angle and a deficiency of columellar show. Progression of the disease often occurs with partial or complete destruction of the nasal bones with resultant flattening of the nasal bridge. In rare cases, scar tissue retraction can lead to virtual elimination of the nasal vestibule, thereby causing significant functional deficits. Fortunately, it is exceedingly rare for the nasal skin–soft tissue envelope to be affected by the disease.

LEPROSY DRUG REGIMEN

Given the significant functional and aesthetic consequences of the lepromatous saddle-nose deformity, patients affected with the disease are often eager to undergo surgical correction. However, it is important that maximal medical management has been employed before operative intervention. In the 1990s, the recommendation for treatment of leprosy by the World Health Organization (WHO) involved 2 years of multidrug therapy (MDT) with rifampicin, dapsone, and clofazimine.[8] More recently, the recommended treatment duration was decreased to 12 months,[9] with the newest recommendations for MDT courses as short as 6 months.[10] Because there is little expert consensus and a dearth of long-term, controlled trials on the length of therapy, the authors of this article recommend ensuring that the patient has received an adequate medication trial while demonstrating no evidence of active lesions or continued mucosal/cartilaginous destruction before initiating operative planning.

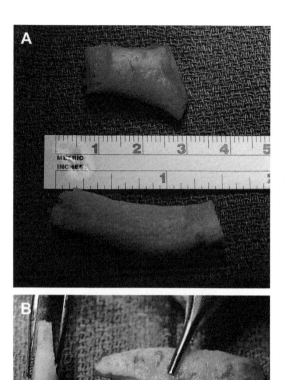

Fig. 2. (*A*) Grafts consisting of costal cartilage and perichondrium from the left seventh and eighth ribs immediately over harvest and (*B*) after carving before placement (dorsal onlay graft (*above*) and columellar strut (*below*)).

LEPROSY SADDLE-NOSE DEFORMITY CORRECTION

Many authors have devised different classification systems for grading saddle-nose deformities to predict operative intervention and/or framework material needed for repair.[3,6,11–13] However, in the published literature for repair of the leprosy saddle-nose, there is a tendency to use only one technique for all repairs based on the surgeon's expertise or preference, or to use various techniques without a description of the indication for each type of repair.[5,14,15] Additionally, there is no consensus on the ideal implant material (ie, autologous costal cartilage, homologous irradiated rib cartilage, auricular cartilage, allografts, or bone) for use in reconstruction of the saddle-nose, because each surgeon tends to hold individual preferences.

AUGMENTATION FOR SEVERE SADDLE-NOSE

Although septal cartilage is seen by many as the ideal grafting material,[16–19] its use is precluded in rebuilding the severe saddle-nose, because there is almost always a deficiency of viable cartilage. Thus, additional sources of grafting material must be used. Irradiated homologous rib cartilage (IHRC) is a practical option with principal

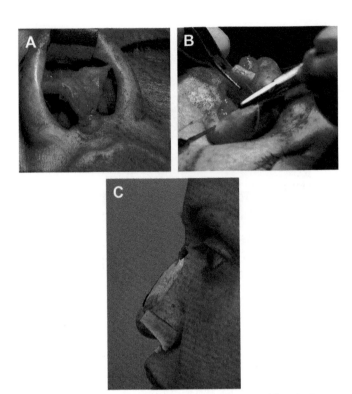

Fig. 3. (*A*) Intraoperative view demonstrating standard open rhinoplasty approach. Note that the patient's lower lateral cartilages have been spared by her infection with *Mycobacterium leprae*. (*B*) Placement of extended columellar strut using multiple, interrupted permanent sutures. (*C*) Photographic illustration of costal cartilage graft placement.

advantages being avoidance of donor-site morbidity and associated perioperative risks, such as pneumothorax. Furthermore, IHRC is associated with low rates of infection and extrusion. However, reports on the resorption rates of IHRC used in rhinoplasty have been inconsistent, with many long-term results showing low or negligible graft-resorption rates[20] while other series demonstrate resorption rates to be much higher.[21,22] In the only published study on IHRC use in rhinoplasty for destructive diseases of the nasal framework, there was significant resorption of the irradiated rib cartilage, which required multiple revision surgeries. The authors therefore recommend against using IHRC in such cases whenever possible.[23]

Recently, Menger and associates[6] described their experience correcting the leprosy-affected nose. They examined their results and experience with over 17 leprosy patients. Using a variety of auricular and costal cartilage grafts, they found that reconstruction of the leprosy nose resulted in satisfactory appearance in almost all cases with autogenous cartilage. Importantly, they found resorption of some of the grafts over a period of time. One can speculate that resorption of costal cartilage in leprosy may be higher than that in standard cases due to poor mucosal blood supply in this subset of patients. In addition, if leprosy is still active, the destructive nature of leprosy can lead to continued destruction of autogenous cartilage.

Alloplastic materials are another viable option for reconstruction of the leprosy saddle-nose. These implants are easy to obtain and easy to use. However, these materials are not biologically incorporated into the host tissue and therefore carry

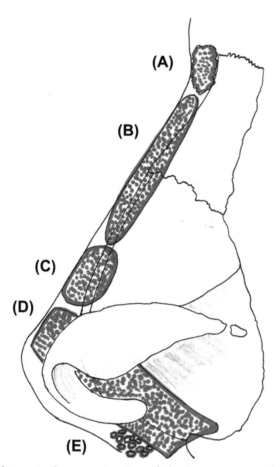

Fig. 4. Diagram demonstrating reconstruction of the Leprosy nose with costal cartilage. Costal perichondrium was placed superiorly for augmentation of patient's radix (A). Dorsal augmentation was achieved by placement of two onlay grafts (B, C). Tip support was reestablished with an extended columellar strut (D), and the premaxilla was enhanced with multiple small pieces of costal cartilage (E).

the highest rates of infection, extrusion, and foreign body reaction of any graft material.[24] In a nose with preexisting chronic inflammation and damaged microvasculature, such as that found in leprosy, the use of an alloplastic material may reignite the inflammatory response, which could result in rejection and injury to the viable soft tissue envelope. Additionally, these grafts primarily provide augmentation rather than structural support during rhinoplasty. In a recent review of the use of polytetrafluoroethylene (PTFE) in rhinoplasty by Godin and colleagues,[25] the authors found a graft infection rate of 3.2% and recommended that PTFE not be used in patients with septal perforations.

In the authors' experience, autologous costal cartilage has proven to be the most reliable material for nasal framework reconstruction when septal cartilage is either unavailable or insufficient. Costal cartilage will supply the surgeon with ample amounts of cartilage to repair any major structural defect, and because it is an autologous graft, there is no host immune response. Therefore, the rates of graft rejection, infection, and extrusion are extremely low.[16,19] One concern with autologous costal cartilage is the theoretical potential for graft resorption. Multiple studies have shown no evidence of resoprtion of costal cartilage grafts when correct surgical technique is used.[17,26] Additionally, Menger and colleagues[6] used autologous costal cartilage to reconstruct the nasal dorsum in 17 patients with saddle-nose deformities caused by leprosy, and noted only one case of complete resorption of the graft after a 2-year follow-up. One author (A.R.S) has used autogenous costal cartilage in over 85 cases, and has noted resorption in one case, after an infection to the nose in an immunocompromised patient. This author has not noted any cases of warping or extrusion during this time.

Another concern with autologous costal cartilage grafts is the potential for warping, which despite careful technique, continues to be the primary problem with the use of autologous rib cartilage.[19] Adams and colleagues[27] recently demonstrated that the warping characteristics of irradiated and nonirrradiated rib cartilage are similar, and recommended the use of IHRC only in cases where autologous cartilage is unavailable or the patient desires avoiding donor site incisions. Meticulous carving techniques, the removal of all perichondrium, and adequate support of the graft are crucial in obtaining desirable results. Additionally, insertion of the graft may be delayed for at least 30 minutes to allow initial warping to occur.

The authors of this study advocate the use of the extended columellar strut rather than the use of a standard columellar strut. An extended columellar strut is used when the septum is missing and/or deficient. In this case, the entire native septum was absent. One common mistake of surgeons using this technique is to make the columellar strut "too wide." Unfortunately, when the columellar strut is excessively wide, the columella will appear wide and often widen the infratip lobule, creating an unrefined look to the nose. One advantage of costal cartilage lies in its strength, obviating the need for excessively wide grafts.

Recreation of the nasal dorsum is a challenge for surgeons. Many surgeons incorporate large costal cartilage pieces onto the nasal dorsum, in an effort to rebuild the nose. However, for most patients with a saddle-nose deformity, the collapse occurs within the cartilaginous portion of the nose. The authors advocate a more technically advanced approach to dorsal augmentation. Rather than excessive augmentation of the nasal bridge, less costal cartilage is placed on the bridge of the nose. In addition, the bony dorsum is gently rasped to accommodate a dorsal graft. Overall, the effort should be to build a natural dorsum, rather than adding excessive bulk to the nasal upper third.

SUMMARY

Despite great advances in medicine, leprosy remains a common granulamatous process within the world. The satisfactory treatment of the saddle-nose created by leprosy can be accomplished by using autogenous cartilage. Additionally, careful technical execution and sound aesthetic judgment are critically important to reconstructing these challenging deformities.

REFERENCES

1. Prevalence of Leprosy. World Health Organization 2008. Available at: www.who. int/lep/en. Accessed May 8, 2009.
2. Britton WJ, Lockwood DNJ. Leprosy. Lancet 2004;363:1209–19.
3. Schwarz RJ, Macdonald M. A rational approach to nasal reconstruction in Leprosy. Plast Reconstr Surg 2003;114(4):876–82.

4. Farina R. Total rhinoplasty for deformities following leprosy. Plast Reconstr Surg 1957;20(1):78–82.
5. Anita NH, Pandya NJ. Surgical treatment of the nasal deformities of leprosy: a 16-year review. Plast Reconstr Surg 1977;60(5):768–77.
6. Menger DJ, Fokkens WJ, Lohuis PJFM, et al. Reconstructive surgery of the leprosy nose: a new approach. J Plast Reconstr Aesthet Surg 2007;60:152–62.
7. Fokkens WJ, Nolst Trenite GJ, Vinmond M, et al. The nose in leprosy: immunohistology of the nasal mucosa. Int J Lepr 1998;66(3):328–39.
8. Chemotherapy of leprosy. Report of a WHO Study Group. World Health Organ Tech Rep Ser 1994;847:1–24.
9. WHO Expert Committee on Leprosy. World Health Organ Tech Rep Ser 1998;874: 1–43.
10. Report on third meeting of the WHO Technical Advisory Group on elimination of leprosy. Geneva: World Health Organization; 2002. Report No. WHO/CDS/CPE/CEE/2002.29.
11. Tardy ME Jr, Schwartz M, Parras G. Saddle nose deformity: autogenous graft repair. Facial Plast Surg 1989;6(2):121–34.
12. Romo T 3rd, Sclafini AP, Sabini P. Reconstruction of the major saddle nose deformity using composite allo-implants. Facial Plast Surg 1998;14(2):151–7.
13. Thomassin JM, Paris J, Richard-Vitton T. Management and aesthetic results of support grafts in saddle nose surgery. Aesthetic Plast Surg 2001;25(5):332–7.
14. Tovey FI. Reconstruction of the nose in leprosy patients. Lepr Rev 1965;36(4): 215–20.
15. Farina R. Total rhinoplasty for the destroyed nose. In: McDowell F, Enna C, editors. Surgical rehabilitation in leprosy. Baltimore (MD): Williams & Wilkins; 1974. p. 143–8.
16. Cardenas-Camarena L, Guerrero MT. Use of cartilaginous autografts in nasal surgery: 8 years of experience. Plast Reconstr Surg 1999;103:1003–14.
17. Collawn SS, Fix J, Moore JR, et al. Nasal cartilage grafts: more than a decade of experience. Plast Reconstr Surg 1997;100:1547–52.
18. Tardy ME, Denneny J, Fritsch MH. The versatile cartilage autograft in reconstruction of the nose and face. Laryngoscope 1985;95:523–33.
19. Lovice DB, Mingrone MD, Toriumi DM. Grafts and implants in rhinoplasty and nasal reconstruction. Otolaryngol Clin North Am 1999;32(1):113–41.
20. Murakami CS, Cook TA, Guida RA. Nasal reconstruction with articulated irradiated rib cartilage. Arch Otolaryngol Head Neck Surg 1991;117:327–30.
21. Welling RO, Maves MD, Schuller DE, et al. Irradiated homologous cartilage grafts: long term results. Arch Otolaryngol Head Neck Surg 1988;114:291–5.
22. Burke AJC, Wang TD, Cook TA. Irradiated homograft rib cartilage in facial reconstruction. Arch Facial Plast Surg 2004;6:334–41.
23. Congdon D, Sherris DA, Specks U, et al. Long-term follow-up of repair of external nasal deformities in patients with Wegener's granulomatosis. Laryngoscope 2002;112(4):731–7.
24. Porter JP. Grafts in rhinoplasty: alloplastic vs. autogenous. Arch Otolaryngol Head Neck Surg 2000;126(4):558–61.
25. Godin MS, Waldman SR, Johnson CM. Nasal augmentation using Gore-tex: a 10-year experience. Arch Facial Plast Surg 1999;1:118–21.
26. Cakmak O, Ergin T. The versatile autogenous costal cartilage graft in septorhioplasty. Arch Facial Plast Surg 2002;4(3):172–6.
27. Adams WP Jr, Rohrich RJ, Gunter JP, et al. The rate of warping in irradiated and nonirradiated homograft rib cartilage: a controlled comparison and clinical implications. Plast Reconstr Surg 1999;103(1):265–70.

A Patient Seeking Aesthetic Revision Rhinoplasty and Correction of Nasal Obstruction

Daniel G. Becker, MD, FACS[a],*, Jason D. Bloom, MD[b], David Gudis, MD[b]

KEYWORDS

- Case study—nasal obstruction • Revision rhinoplasty
- Nasal obstruction • Nasal valve collapse • Inferior turbinate
- Endoscopic septoplasty

CASE REPORT

A 57-year-old white female patient presented for consultation for improvement in her aesthetic nasal appearance and also for evaluation and treatment of nasal obstruction. She had a past history of external septorhinoplasty. She had no allergy symptoms and, in fact, had been tested for environmental allergies by her family doctor by a modified radioallergosorbent test (mRAST) blood test and was negative for significant allergies. She reported bilateral nasal obstruction. She was questioned about other related symptoms; she denied facial pain or pressure, but she did report recurrent sinus infections and postnasal drainage. She denied Afrin use. She did not smoke. She reported persistent nasal obstruction and persistent sinus symptoms despite the use of over-the-counter medications, such as oral decongestants, antihistamines, mucolytics, and saline nasal spray. She also reported no benefit from nasal steroid sprays or other prescription medications.

Physical examination revealed alar retraction and nasal valve collapse. She had middle vault collapse with an inverted V abnormality as well. A modified Cottle maneuver resulted in partial improvement of her nasal obstruction. Anterior rhinoscopy revealed normal inferior turbinates and a left deviated septum. Topical anesthesia with Afrin and Pontocaine was followed by rigid nasal endoscopy. This

[a] Division of Facial Plastic and Reconstructive Surgery, Department of Otorhinolaryngology, University of Pennsylvania Hospital, Becker Nose and Sinus Center, LLC, 400 Medical Center Drive, Suite B, Sewell, NJ 08080, USA
[b] Department of Otorhinolaryngology, University of Pennsylvania Hospital, Philadelphia, PA, USA
* Corresponding author.
E-mail address: beckermailbox@aol.com (D.G. Becker).

Otolaryngol Clin N Am 42 (2009) 557–565
doi:10.1016/j.otc.2009.03.001
0030-6665/09/$ – see front matter © 2009 Published by Elsevier Inc.

revealed a leftward deviated septum causing significant nasal obstruction. Superiorly, at the point of maximal deviation, the nasal endoscope could not be passed on the left. The endoscope could be passed along the floor of the nose only on the left. On the right, examination was notable for an enlarged middle turbinate. There were small left unilateral polyps in the middle meatus but no other masses or concerning lesions. The nasopharynx was clear.

A coronal sinus CT scan was obtained (**Fig. 1**). This revealed the deviated septum, a markedly enlarged and aerated middle turbinate (concha bullosa), and evidence of chronic sinusitis.

The patient underwent revision external septorhinoplasty, endoscopic sinus surgery, and ear cartilage harvest for cartilage grafting. She underwent bilateral placement of spreader grafts, bilateral alar batten graft placement, and aesthetic corrections as well. At the time of surgery, the surgeon was prepared to undertake endoscopic revision septoplasty if necessary, but it was noted that a thorough septoplasty had been performed. A large portion of the septum was membranous only, without intervening cartilage or bone. On excision of the lateral aspect of the concha bullosa, the deviated septum straightened because it was apparently being held leftward by the large concha bullosa (**Fig. 2**). After surgery, the patient reported resolution of her nasal obstruction without the need for medical therapy. She was also pleased with her aesthetic appearance 1 year after surgery. **Fig. 3** shows the patient preoperatively and **Fig. 4** show the patient 1 year postoperatively.

DISCUSSION
Nasal Obstruction Differential Diagnosis

It is important to keep in mind the differential diagnosis of conditions causing nasal obstruction when treating patients with this complaint (**Box 1**). In the senior author's rhinoplasty practice, problems causing nasal obstruction have included chronic sinusitis with and without polyps, deviated septum, inferior and middle turbinate hypertrophy, adenoid hypertrophy, tumors, concha bullosa, internal and external valve collapse, and other conditions.[1]

Nasal Obstruction History and Physical Examination

A detailed history and physical examination, including intranasal examination with and without topicalization with a decongestant and nasal endoscopy, are critical aspects in the evaluation and treatment of every patient presenting with a complaint of nasal obstruction. In patients seeking rhinoplasty, the history should elicit the presence of nasal obstruction, chronic or recurrent sinusitis, postnasal drip and cough, facial

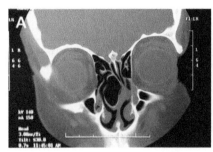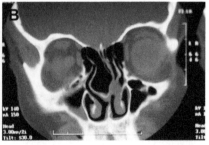

Fig. 1. (*A, B*) CT scans demonstrate deviated septum, large concha bullosa, and evidence of chronic sinusitis.

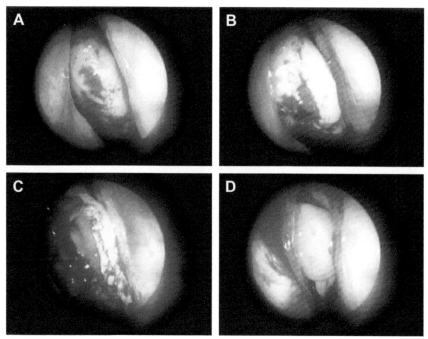

Fig. 2. (*A*) Intraoperative view of concha bullosa. The concha bullosa is incised (*B*), and the lateral aspect is excised with through-biting forceps, preserving the medial aspect (*C*). (*D*) On the left side in this patient, polyps were notable and were addressed.

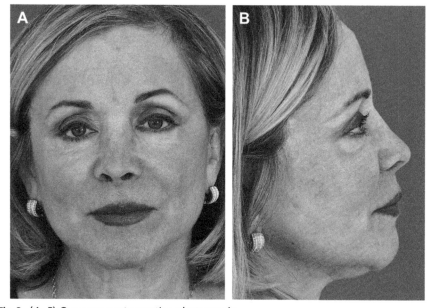

Fig. 3. (*A, B*) One-year postoperative photographs.

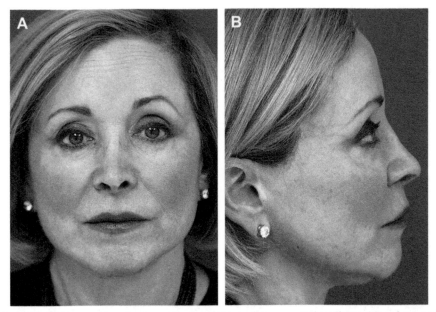

Fig. 4. (A, B) Preoperative photographs of a patient who requested aesthetic rhinoplasty and functional nasal improvement.

Box 1
Differential diagnosis for nasal obstruction
Allergic rhinitis
Rhinosinusitis
Rhinitis medicamentosa
Atrophic rhinitis
Deviated septum
Nasal valve collapse
Nasal polyps
Adenoid hypertrophy
Choanal atresia
Nasal tumors
Inferior turbinate hypertrophy
Middle turbinate hypertrophy
Viral infection (upper respiratory infection)
Septal hematoma
Septal abscess
Nasal foreign body
Overresection or overnarrowing after osteotomies

pressure or pain, ear pressure or pain, hearing loss, loss of sense of smell or taste, halitosis, and other pertinent findings.[1–7] A history of prior sinus surgery, rhinoplasty, or other nasal surgery should be noted. The patient should be questioned and, when appropriate, evaluated for allergies.[1–4,7]

All medications taken, including aspirin and aspirin-containing products and herbal medicines, such as gingko biloba, that can increase intraoperative bleeding, should be carefully recorded. A history of topical nasal decongestant abuse may lead to the diagnosis and treatment of rhinitis medicamentosa.

External nasal examination is important in all patients with nasal obstruction. Internal and external nasal valve collapse should be recognized when present. A narrow middle third of the nose may be an indication of internal nasal valve compromise.[5,6,8–12] The Cottle maneuver may be helpful in the identification of internal nasal valve collapse. The classic description of this maneuver involves pulling the cheek laterally, resulting in improved nasal breathing. Lateralizing the cheek secondarily moves the nasal soft tissue and widens the nasal valve. A more direct approach is to lateralize the nasal soft tissue gently using a small curette or other straight probe. This must be done before topicalization. Improvement of nasal breathing after minimal (1–2 mm) lateralization of the nasal sidewall suggests that nasal valve abnormality contributes to nasal obstruction. There is the possibility of a false-positive result with this test; thus, the surgeon must be careful to lateralize the nasal sidewall in a realistic manner.[5,6,8–12]

External nasal valve collapse also should be recognized when present. Evidence of prior nasal surgery with excessive reduction and narrowing of the internal and external nasal valve may be immediately evident or it may be subtle.[5,6,13]

Intranasal examination should be performed before and after topicalization with a vasoconstricting agent. When indicated by the patient history or by findings on anterior rhinoscopy, a nasal endoscopic examination is also performed. Abnormalities not appreciated on rhinoscopy may be noted on careful endoscopy by a skilled endoscopist in the office after appropriate topicalization and may be of great use in identifying physical findings.[1,14,15]

Nasal Obstruction Imaging

In this setting, the physician may also consider obtaining a coronal sinus CT scan, especially in the patient with a history of chronic nasal obstruction. Chronic nasal obstruction is the most common presenting symptom of anterior ethmoid sinus disease. A CT scan may demonstrate evidence of chronic sinusitis, including obstruction of the osteomeatal complex or the presence of polyps, and also of other causes of nasal obstruction, such as concha bullosa or a posterior septal deviation, which may occasionally be unappreciated without an endoscopic examination or CT scan.

Nasal Obstruction Endoscopic Examination

Levine[14] reported that 39% of patients with a complaint of nasal obstruction had findings on endoscopic examination that were not identified with traditional rhinoscopy. Many of Levine's patients had seen other physicians for this problem and had not received appropriate treatment.

Lanfranchi and colleagues[15] reported on the importance of diagnostic nasal endoscopy in patients with nasal obstruction who present for septorhinoplasty. In their report, a retrospective chart review was undertaken on all patients presenting to the senior author from April 1997 through July 1999 for septorhinoplasty who reported a history of nasal obstruction. Patients seeking cosmetic rhinoplasty without functional complaint were excluded from the study. All patients requesting septorhinoplasty who complained of any degree of nasal obstruction underwent nasal endoscopy. In some cases, a CT scan was additionally undertaken. Findings identified by anterior rhinoscopy were recorded, and additional findings not identified on anterior rhinoscopy were recorded. Ninety-five patients, including 83 undergoing primary rhinoplasty and 12 undergoing revision rhinoplasty, were included in the study.

Nasal examination, including anterior rhinoscopy, revealed obstruction attributable to a deviated septum, nasal valve compromise, and inferior turbinate hypertrophy. Nasal endoscopy revealed additional pathologic findings, including obstructing adenoids, enlarged middle turbinates with concha bullosa, choanal stenosis, nasal polyps, and chronic sinusitis refractory to medical therapy. Additional surgical therapy was undertaken in 28 patients because of findings on endoscopic examination (nine patients underwent partial middle turbinectomy for concha bullosa, 13 underwent endoscopic sinus surgery, two required adenoidectomy, one underwent repair of nasal stenosis, and three required endoscopic septoplasty for persisting posterior septal deviation despite prior septal surgery).

Based on these results, the senior author recommends that patients presenting for septorhinoplasty who note nasal obstruction should undergo anterior rhinoscopy followed by nasal endoscopy. In a significant number of patients (such as the one presented here), nasal endoscopy allows identification of clinically significant pathologic findings and thereby alters surgical therapy.[15]

SPECIFIC CAUSES OF NASAL OBSTRUCTION IN THIS CASE STUDY
Middle Turbinates

Airway blockage may be partially attributable to enlargement of the middle turbinates (especially with a concha bullosa) (see **Fig. 2**). Concha bullosa may be found in up to 10% of individuals. Middle turbinate hypertrophy attributable to a concha bullosa may contribute to nasal obstruction and may be corrected by conservative partial middle turbinectomy, which can cause an improvement of airflow and a significant decrease in nasal resistance.[16] Resection of the lateral aspect of the concha is typically performed under endoscopic guidance to allow for precise excision and may significantly relieve nasal obstruction.

In patients with a deviated septum, return of the septum to midline by means of septoplasty may actually diminish the airway on the side of a hypertrophied middle turbinate (**Fig. 5**). Partial sacrifice of an enlarged turbinate in this situation may significantly contribute to improvement in nasal breathing.[16]

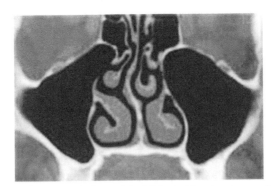

Fig. 5. This CT scan suggests that a left partial middle turbinectomy may also be warranted in this patient, because straightening the septum would narrow the left nasal passage.

Septum

Deviation of the nasal septum is a common cause of nasal obstruction. The contribution of a deviated septum to nasal obstruction may be addressed by straightening it by means of septoplasty. Identification of the anatomic cause of the deviation helps to guide surgical treatment. Typically, a stepwise graduated approach is advisable.[5]

Certain abnormalities of the septum warrant special attention. The persistent posterior septal deviation after prior septoplasty is a unique challenge that can be addressed by endoscopic septoplasty.[17–22]

Endoscopic Septoplasty

Endoscopic septoplasty is a well-described technique for correction of septal deformities.[17–22] First described in 1991,[17] its use has been reported for the treatment of isolated septal spurs[17–22] and in the treatment of more broad-based septal deformities.[21] Advantages of the endoscopic technique include potentially improved visualization of posterior septal deformities, the opportunity for limited minimally invasive procedures, and potential improved access in certain revision cases.

Endoscopic septoplasty is useful in difficult revision nasal surgeries (septoplasty and septorhinoplasty) in which persisting obstructing septal deviation persists despite prior septoplasty. Although septoplasty and septorhinoplasty do not commonly require endoscopic approaches, the endoscopic approach may be a useful adjunct in difficult revision cases in which complete elevation of a mucoperichondrial flap presents difficulties. Examples include a persistent posterior septal obstruction after prior septoplasty or after septal injury (eg, hematoma, abscess) with loss of cartilaginous septum. In these cases, typical surgical dissection planes are obliterated and complete elevation of a mucoperichondrial or mucoperiosteal flap may be difficult. The ability to bypass these adherent areas and to address a persisting deviation directly, elevating the mucosal flap directly over the offending deviation using endoscopic techniques, greatly facilitates treatment.

If an isolated posterior deformity is addressed, the more anterior mucosa is bypassed and the mucoperichondrium is incised just anterior to the offending cartilage or bone. Mucoperichondrial and mucoperiosteal flap elevation proceeds and may be facilitated by a suction elevator. The cartilage or bone is incised several millimeters posterior to the mucosal incision, and the contralateral mucosal flap is elevated. Deviated portions of septal cartilage and bone are corrected or removed. Straightened or morselized cartilage may be replaced, and the septal flaps may be closed with a quilting suture, although in more limited cases, suturing may not be necessary.

Nasal Valve Collapse

Nasal valve problems and their treatment are well described.[1,5,6,8–13,23–26] Evaluation and treatment of these complex problems require a thorough understanding of the anatomy and physiology of the nasal valve. Even when the surgeon has ascertained that nasal valve problems are contributory to nasal obstruction, further evaluation is advisable to assess other possible causes. Otherwise, the surgeon and patient may be frustrated when nasal obstruction persists despite surgical treatment.

Chronic Sinusitis

The evaluation and treatment of sinusitis have been thoroughly described in the medical literature.[3,4,27–29] Although sinusitis most commonly presents with several symptoms, including nasal obstruction, it is notable that nasal obstruction is the most common symptom of anterior ethmoid disease.[3,4] When performed simultaneously, these operations can be performed by the same surgeon, as in the case described in this article, or they can be performed using a two-team approach.[30] The literature has been supportive of concurrent rhinoplasty and sinus surgery when the sinus surgery and the rhinoplasty are of moderate severity or complexity.[3,30–34]

SUMMARY

In this patient seeking cosmetic revision rhinoplasty, causes of nasal obstruction included nasal valve collapse, deviated septum, concha bullosa, and chronic sinusitis with polyps. Thorough evaluation, including nasal endoscopy and a CT scan, was necessary to guide proper diagnosis and treatment. This patient seeking aesthetic and functional improvement is therefore illustrative of the need for a thorough evaluation of a patient presenting with nasal obstruction. The rhinoplasty surgeon should be aware of the differential diagnosis of nasal obstruction and should proceed with thorough evaluation or refer the patient for appropriate complete evaluation.

REFERENCES

1. Becker DG. Septoplasty and turbinate surgery. Aesthet Surg J 2003;23:393–403.
2. Jafek BW, Dodson BT. Nasal obstruction. In: Bailey, editor. Head and neck surgery— otolaryngology. 2nd edition. Philadelphia: Lippincott-Raven; 1998. p. 371–97.
3. Becker DG, Kennedy DW. Indications for sinus surgery in patients undergoing rhinoplasty. Aesthetic Plast Surg 1998;18:129–31.
4. Senior B, Kennedy DW. Endoscopic sinus surgery: a review. Otolaryngol Clin North Am 1997;30:313–30.
5. Tardy ME. Rhinoplasty: the art and the science. Philadelphia: WB Saunders Company; 1997.
6. Tardy ME, Toriumi DM. Philosophy and principles of rhinoplasty. In: Papel ID, Nachlas NE, editors. Facial plastic and reconstructive surgery. St. Louis (MO): Mosby; 1990. p. 278–94.
7. Mabry RL. Allergy for rhinologists. Otolaryngol Clin North Am 1998;31:175–88.
8. Toriumi DM. Management of the middle nasal vault in rhinoplasty. Operat Tech Plast Reconstr Surg 1995;2:16–30.
9. Constantian MB, Clardy RB. The relative importance of septal and nasal valvular surgery in correcting airway obstruction in primary and secondary rhinoplasty. Plast Reconstr Surg 1996;98:38–54.
10. Sheen JH. Spreader graft: a method of reconstructing the roof of the middle nasal vault following rhinoplasty. Plast Reconstr Surg 1984;73:230–7.
11. Goode RL. Surgery of the incompetent nasal valve. Laryngoscope 1985;95: 546–55.
12. Johnson CM, Toriumi DM. Open structure rhinoplasty. Philadelphia: Saunders; 1990.
13. Constantian MB. The incompetent external nasal valve: pathophysiology and treatment in primary and secondary rhinoplasty. Plast Reconstr Surg 1994;93: 919–31.
14. Levine HL. The office diagnosis of nasal and sinus disorders using rigid nasal endoscopy. Otolaryngol Head Neck Surg 1990;102:370–3.
15. Lanfranchi PV, Steiger J, Sparano A, et al. Diagnostic and surgical endoscopy in functional septorhinoplasty. Facial Plast Surg 2004;20:207–15.
16. Cook PR, Begegni A, Bryant C, et al. Effect of partial middle turbinectomy on nasal airflow and resistance. Otolaryngol Head Neck Surg 1995;113:413–9.

17. Lanza DC, Kennedy DW, Zinreich SJ. Nasal endoscopy and its surgical applications. In: Lee KJ, editor. Essential otolaryngology: head and neck surgery. 5th edition. New York: Medical Examination Publ Co; 1991. p. 373–87.
18. Lanza DC, Rosin DF, Kennedy DW. Endoscopic septal spur resection. Am J Rhinol 1993;7:213–6.
19. Cantrell H. Limited septoplasty for endoscopic sinus surgery. Otolaryngol Head Neck Surg 1997;116:274–7.
20. Giles WC, Gross CW, Abram AC, et al. Endoscopic septoplasty. Laryngoscope 1994;104:1507–9.
21. Hwang PH, McLaughlin RB, Lanza DC, et al. Endoscopic septoplasty: indications, technique, and results. Otolaryngol Head Neck Surg 1999;120:678–82.
22. Becker DG. Endoscopic septoplasty in functional septorhinoplasty. Operat Otolaryngol Head Neck Surg 2000.
23. Toriumi DM, Josen J, Weinberger MS, et al. Use of alar batten grafts for correction of nasal valve collapse. Arch Otolaryngol Head Neck Surg 1997;123:802–8.
24. Toriumi DM, Becker DG. Rhinoplasty dissection manual. Philadelphia: Lippincott, Williams & Wilkins; 1999.
25. Becker DG. My personal approach and philosophy. In: Becker DG, editor. Revision rhinoplasty. New York; 2008. p. 189–201.
26. Becker DG. Treatment of nasal obstruction from nasal valve collapse with alar batten grafts. J Long Term Eff Med Implants 2003;13:259–69.
27. Lanza DC, Kennedy DW. Adult rhinosinusitis defined. (Report of the Rhinosinusitis Task Force Committee Meeting). Otolaryngol Head Neck Surg 1997;117 (3 Pt 2):S1–7.
28. Hadley JA, Schaefer SD. Clinical evaluation of rhinosinusitis: history and physical examination. (Report of the Rhinosinusitis Task Force Committee Meeting). Otolaryngol Head Neck Surg 1997;117(3 Pt 2):S8–11.
29. Becker DG, Kennedy DW. Functional endoscopic sinus surgery: a review. Russian J Rhinol 1998;1:4–14.
30. Marcus B, Patel Z, Busquets J, et al. The utility of concurrent rhinoplasty and sinus surgery: a 2-team approach. Arch Facial Plast Surg 2006;8:260–2.
31. Gliklich RE, Lauretano AM. The risk of nasal osteotomies after ethmoid sinus surgery. Arch Otolaryngol Head Neck Surg 1995;121:1315–8.
32. Nachlas NE. Endoscopic sinus surgery as an adjunct to rhinoplasty. In: Papel ID, Nachlas NE, editors. Facial plastic and reconstructive surgery. Philadelphia: Mosby Year Book; 1992. p. 350–9.
33. Toffel PH. Simultaneous secure endoscopic sinus surgery and rhinoplasty. Ear Nose Throat J 1994;73:554–6, 558–60, 565.
34. Rizk SS, Edelstein DR, Matarasso A. Concurrent functional endoscopic sinus surgery and rhinoplasty. Ann Plast Surg 1997;38:323–9.

Treatment of Nasal Obstruction in the Posttraumatic Nose

Christina L. Corey, MD, Sam P. Most, MD*

KEYWORDS
- Nasal obstruction • Nasal deformity • Trauma • Nasal trauma
- Rhinoplasty

The nose is considered the most prominent feature of the face. As a result, fractures of the nose and nasal region account for approximately half of all facial fractures.[1–3] The sequelae of trauma to the nose include nasal deformity and nasal obstruction that can have a long-term negative impact on patient quality of life and thus often require repair. According to Rohrich and Adams, 40% to 42% of patients after nasal trauma have significant septal deformities that require subsequent septorhinoplasty.[1] This article focuses on the treatment of nasal obstruction in the posttraumatic nose. Nasal obstruction following trauma is a complex problem that poses several challenges for the facial plastic surgeon. Successful management of posttraumatic nasal obstruction relies on careful analysis and accurate diagnosis. Treatment of the posttraumatic nose must balance the seemingly disparate goals of re-establishing structure, improving contour and esthetics, and restoring the nasal airway.

ETIOLOGY

Trauma to the nose is most often sustained in fights (34%), accidents (28%), and sports (23%).[3,4] Frontal force causes damage ranging from simple fracture of the nasal bones to severe flattening of the nasal bones and septum. Splaying of the nasal bones with widening of the nasal width may also occur. Lateral force may depress only one nasal bone; however, with sufficient force, both bones may be displaced. In addition, lateral force can cause severe septal displacement, which can further twist or buckle the nose.[5] Septal fragments may overlap, creating further difficulty in reduction. Furthermore, a C-shaped deformity may occur. This defect usually begins under the dorsum of the nose, extends posteriorly and inferiorly through the perpendicular plate of the ethmoid, and ends with an anterior curve in the cartilaginous septum approximately 1 cm above the maxillary crest.[5] Superior-directed force is rare and may cause

Division of Facial Plastic & Reconstructive Surgery, Department of Otolaryngology-Head and Neck Surgery, Stanford University School of Medicine, 801 Welch Road, Stanford, CA 94305, USA
* Corresponding author.
E-mail address: smost@ohns.stanford.edu (S.P. Most).

Otolaryngol Clin N Am 42 (2009) 567–578
doi:10.1016/j.otc.2009.03.002

severe septal fractures and dislocation of the quadrangular cartilage. With the increasing use of air bags in automobiles, a shift in the mechanism of injury and the type of nasal fractures has occurred, resulting in an increase in the incidence of septal injury in nasal fractures without concurrent nasal bone fracture.[4]

ANALYSIS OF THE POSTTRAUMA NOSE

The cornerstone of a thorough analysis is a detailed history with particular attention to the type, date, and frequency of traumatic events as well as any previous surgeries. Even seemingly minor trauma early in life can produce a delayed marked deformity not manifesting itself until the nose and face grow significantly at puberty.[6–8] The date of trauma and any past surgeries is important because it may influence the timing of any further surgery that may be required. Although closed reduction of nasal bone fractures may be performed either within the first several hours following injury before the development of significant edema or between 4 to 7 days following the injury after the resolution of facial edema, an open approach is often required if nasal obstruction is to be adequately addressed in addition to nasal deformity. In these cases, a delay of 6 to 12 months after injury is often required to allow fractures to stabilize and wounds to heal before surgical correction of nasal obstruction or deformity. Patients who have sustained multiple traumas or have had previous nasal surgery may not only be more complex but may also lack any usable septal cartilage grafts. As a result, it is important to ask patients about any prior history of nasal surgery or pre-injury septal deviation. In addition, it is critical to ask patients about the existence of any pre-injury/presurgery nasal obstruction, because they may have underlying unrecognized deviation of the septum or untreated allergic rhinitis or other medical conditions.

A thorough examination is crucial to identifying causes of nasal obstruction in the posttraumatic patient before and after topical decongestion. Anterior rhinoscopy is a valuable tool for assessing the patient. In addition, nasal endoscopy can be useful in the evaluation of patients with posttraumatic nasal obstruction. In a study of 96 consecutive patients undergoing rhinoplasty, preoperative endoscopy identified pathology that required additional surgery in 28 patients, including concha bullosa, posterior septal deviation, adenoid hypertrophy, choanal atresia, and intranasal tumor.[9] The physical examination should be carefully performed, starting with inspection of the septal mucosa for inflammation or other mucosal disease. The septum should also be examined for tears, synechiae, and evidence of septal fractures or perforations. The septum should be evaluated for any deviation, particularly high dorsal or caudal deflection. The presence of turbinate hypertrophy should be noted. In addition, careful attention should be paid to patency of the external nasal valve by identifying any vestibular stenosis, tip ptosis, collapse of the lower lateral cartilages, or nasal muscle deficiency. Furthermore, the zones and grade, as described by Most, of any external nasal valve collapse should be noted.[10] Most categorizes external nasal valve collapse into two zones. Zone 1 is the upper lateral cartilage complex, whereas zone 2 is at or below the junction between the upper and lower lateral cartilages.[10] Collapse at these zones is graded as a percentage of airway closure between the lateral nasal wall and the septum; grade 1 is 0% to 33%, grade 2 is 33% to 66%, and grade 3 is 66% to 100%.[10]

The internal nasal valve should be examined for patency by analyzing the nasal valve area including the nasal septum, upper and lower lateral cartilages (in particular, inferomedial displacement of the upper lateral cartilage), adjacent fibrofatty tissue, piriform aperture, head of the inferior turbinate, and floor of the nose. A diagnosis can be made based on direct inspection of valvular support during quiet and forced inspiration without the distortion induced by a nasal speculum. Collapse of the internal nasal valve can be attributed to medialization of the caudal margin of the upper lateral cartilages due to negative pressure created on inspiration through the nose; these patients typically have pinching or medial collapse of the supra-alar region. The Cottle maneuver is often used to assess internal nasal valve competence. In patients with internal valve collapse, there is often improvement in nasal breathing with lateral retraction of the ipsilateral cheek skin. A modified Cottle maneuver can also be performed with a cotton-tip swab placed intranasally to support the internal nasal valve to determine specifically if improvement in nasal airflow results.

TREATMENT OF POSTTRAUMATIC NASAL OBSTRUCTION

Careful planning is critical to successful treatment of posttraumatic nasal obstruction. Dividing the nose into horizontal thirds assists in preoperative analysis as well as surgical treatment to re-establish structure, improve contour and esthetics, and restore the nasal airway.

Upper Third of Nose

The upper third of the nose consists of the nasal bones, nasal process of the frontal bone, and frontal process of the maxilla. Osteotomies are often employed in rhinoplasty to close an open nasal vault, to narrow the nasal dorsum, or to straighten a deviation in the nasal dorsum.[11,12] Lateral osteotomies are performed in a high-low-high fashion, starting at the anterior end of the inferior turbinate perpendicular to the edge of the piriform aperture and curved anteriorly and superiorly in the nasofacial groove toward the medial canthus (**Fig. 1**). Next, either a superior back fracture, accomplished by turning the osteotome and applying digital pressure, or a superior percutaneous transverse osteotomy is performed. Medial osteotomies are performed between the nasal bones and the septum and angulated superiorly to join the superior

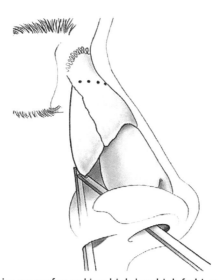

Fig. 1. Lateral osteotomies are performed in a high-low-high fashion, starting at the anterior end of the inferior turbinate perpendicular to the edge of the piriform aperture and curved anteriorly and superiorly in the nasofacial groove toward the medial canthus. (*From* Most SP, Murakami CS. A modern approach to nasal osteotomies. Facial Plast Surg Clin North Am 2005;13(1):88; with permission.)

osteotomy or back-fractured site (**Fig. 2**). When one sidewall is significantly longer than the other, intermediate osteotomies may also be used. Intermediate osteotomies are performed prior with their path parallel to lateral osteotomies, because the former are difficult once the nasal bone is mobilized (**Fig. 3**). In the context of the posttraumatic nose, osteotomies can be used to expand the nasal airway as well as restore the nasal contour of the twisted or deviated nose. When used to address the nasal airway, lateral push-out osteotomies followed by medial osteotomies are used to accommodate a spreader graft and widen the airway. When used to correct deflection of the bony vault, sequential osteotomies are performed from lateral to medial starting on the concave side, often likened to turning the pages of an open book (**Fig. 4**). Using this technique, the concave side is first mobilized to create sufficient space to reposition the deviated structures.

Middle Third of Nose

Treatment of deformities of the middle third is critical to improving the nasal airway. The middle third of the nose includes the upper lateral cartilages, septum, and piriform aperture. Septal pathology may involve cartilage, bone, or both. The septum may be thickened, twisted, scarred, deflected off the maxillary crest, have spurs, or be affected by a combination of these problems. Deviation of the septum secondary to septal fracture or pre-existing septal deflection exacerbated by trauma can often be treated with septoplasty. Convexity or concavity of the septal cartilage can be treated by scoring, crushing, or removal with or without replacement of crushed cartilage between the mucopericondrial flaps. High septal or dorsal deflections may be addressed via an external approach. In addition, inferior turbinate hypertrophy should also be addressed in the treatment of posttraumatic nasal obstruction. Patients with septal deviation have pre-existing turbinate hypertrophy; the inferior turbinate contralateral to the direction of septal deflection is the larger turbinate. Often, turbinate

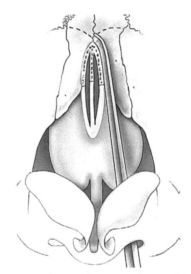

Fig. 2. Medial osteotomies are performed between the nasal bones and the septum and angulated superiorly to join the superior osteotomy or back-fractured site. (*From* Most SP, Murakami CS. A modern approach to nasal osteotomies. Facial Plast Surg Clin North Am 2005;13(1):90; with permission.)

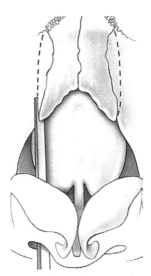

Fig. 3. Intermediate osteotomies are performed prior and with their path parallel to lateral osteotomies, because the former are difficult once the nasal bone is mobilized, when one nasal bone is longer than the other. (*From* Most SP, Murakami CS. A modern approach to nasal osteotomies. Facial Plast Surg Clin North Am 2005;13(1):90; with permission.)

reduction is necessary to mobilize the septum back to the midline. There are many different techniques of turbinate reduction, including monopolar or bipolar cautery, radiofrequency ablation, submucous resection of bone and soft tissue, and partial inferior turbinectomy. Following reduction, the turbinate is then out-fractured laterally.

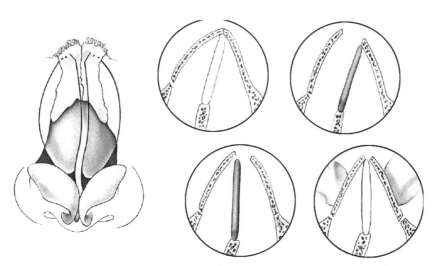

Fig. 4. Sequential osteotomies are performed from lateral to medial starting on the concave side, often likened to turning the pages of an open book. The concave side is first mobilized to create sufficient space to reposition the deviated structures. (*From* Most SP, Murakami CS. A modern approach to nasal osteotomies. Facial Plast Surg Clin North Am 2005;13(1):91; with permission.)

Internal valve insufficiency is caused variably by a narrow angle between the upper lateral cartilage and the septum, deviation of the septum, or enlargement of the anterior portion of the inferior turbinate. Treatment of internal valve insufficiency is critical to improve nasal obstruction in the posttraumatic nose. One must counsel patients that many of the techniques used to address nasal obstruction caused by abnormalities of the internal valve may change the appearance of the nose by widening it. Several techniques have been used to correct internal nasal valve collapse; these techniques are focused on repositioning of the upper lateral cartilage or the addition of structural grafts to support the lateral wall of the nose. The traditional technique used to address internal nasal valve collapse has been the placement of spreader grafts via an endonasal or external approach.[13–15] These grafts are designed to lateralize the upper lateral cartilage by the width of the graft, thereby increasing the cross-sectional area of the nasal valve. Septal, conchal, costal, or cadaveric cartilage, bone, or even Medpor may be used as potential sources for spreader grafts.[15–18] The grafts, typically 1 to 2 mm thick spanning the length of the upper lateral cartilage, are placed in a submucosal pocket between the septum and upper lateral cartilage and fixed in place with one or two horizontal mattress sutures (**Fig. 5**).[15,18] Studies have shown that spreader grafts are effective in treating nasal obstruction due to internal nasal valve narrowing.[19,20] A variation of this technique involves use of the upper lateral cartilages as autospreaders.[21] After dorsal hump reduction, spreader grafts are often required to maintain the internal nasal valve angle. The bony and cartilaginous hump is removed, taking care to preserve the upper lateral cartilages and mucopericondrium. The overprojecting portion of the upper lateral cartilages is then rotated medially to lie between the septum and the medial edge of the upper lateral cartilages (**Fig. 6**). The new dorsal edges of the upper lateral cartilages are then sutured to the rotated autospreader cartilages and secured along the septum.

Alternative techniques in the repair of a narrowed internal nasal valve include dorsal onlay grafts, flaring sutures, and alar batten grafts. Dorsal onlay grafts employ a single piece of cartilage placed over the nose, from bony nasal dorsum to the anterior septal angle, and sutured laterally to each upper lateral cartilage to open the nasal valve. Dorsal onlay grafts are often used to correct severe middle nasal vault deformity and resultant airway problems, particularly in saddle nose deformities.[22] Constantian and Clardy evaluated and compared the efficacy of spreader grafts and dorsal grafts in supporting the internal valves and noted that they were equally effective.[19] In addition, placement of a flaring suture is a method of improving the internal nasal valve angle directly and usually follows the placement of spreader grafts.[18,23] It consists of a mattress suture placed through each upper lateral cartilage and over the dorsum.[18,23] As the suture is tightened, both upper lateral cartilages are pulled dorsally, resulting in a "flaring" action which directly widens the internal nasal valve angle.

The use of alar batten grafts is not only effective for the correction of internal valve collapse but also effective in treating external nasal valve collapse.[8,18] The primary purpose of batten grafts is to reinforce areas of the lateral nasal wall or the alar lobule that collapse secondary to the negative force associated with inspiration. They are placed into a precise pocket at the point of maximal lateral wall collapse, most often using either septal or conchal cartilage as sources of graft materials. For internal nasal valve collapse, battens are typically placed in a pocket at the site of supra-alar collapse and are usually near the caudal margin of the upper lateral cartilage (**Fig. 7**). When external nasal valve collapse is treated, the grafts are typically placed into a pocket caudal to the lateral crura. Batten grafts are wider laterally toward the piriform aperture, to provide maximal structural support, and thin with beveled edges,

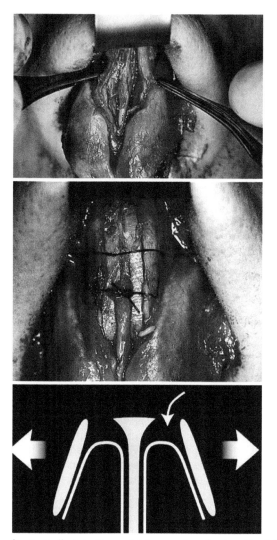

Fig. 5. Spreader grafts, typically 1 to 2 mm thick spanning the length of the upper lateral cartilage, are placed in a submucosal pocket between the septum and the upper lateral cartilage and fixed in place with one or two horizontal mattress sutures to widen the narrowed internal nasal valve. (*From* Schlosser RJ, Park SS. Surgery for the dysfunctional nasal valve. Arch Facial Plast Surg 1999;1:107; with permission.)

especially along the medial aspect of the graft, to minimize cosmetic distortion. The support and stabilization of the lateral nasal wall increases the internal diameter of the nasal airway, thereby increasing dynamic nasal airflow. In a 46-patient review, Toriumi and colleagues[24] concluded that alar batten grafts are effective for long-term correction of internal and external nasal valve collapse in patients who do not have intranasal scarring in the region of the nasal valve, loss of vestibular skin, or excessive narrowing at the piriform aperture.

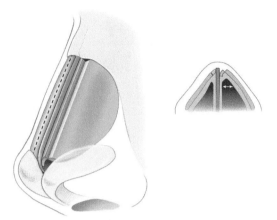

Fig. 6. A variation of the spreader graft technique involves use of the upper lateral cartilages as autospreaders. Following dorsal hump reduction, the overprojecting portions of the upper lateral cartilages are rotated medially to lie between the septum and the medial edge of the upper lateral cartilages.

Lower Third of Nose

Treatment of the posttraumatic nose must also address nasal obstruction due to the structures that comprise the lower third. The lower third of the nose consists of the caudal septum, nasal spine, and medial, middle, and lateral crura of the lower lateral cartilages. In posttraumatic patients, the external valve may be narrowed secondary to the formation of hypertrophic webs; however, more often, wound contracture causes a cicatricial narrowing. In these patients, treatment of nasal obstruction will also treat esthetic issues. As the external valve is widened to re-establish its function in breathing, an improvement will also occur in its appearance and contour. Small webs in the external valve area may be divided primarily and then stented.[25] Repair of more extensive external valve stenosis secondary to cicatrix requires use of primary resection, Z-plasty, full-thickness skin grafts, or composite grafts.

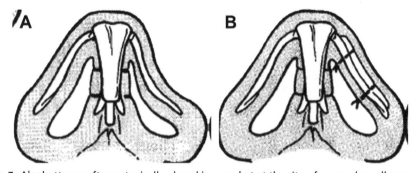

Fig. 7. Alar batten grafts are typically placed in a pocket at the site of supra-alar collapse and are usually near the caudal margin of the upper lateral cartilage. (*A*) Weakness in the lateral crura of the lower lateral cartilage causes alar concavity and narrowing of the nasal airway. (*B*) The support and stabilization of the lateral nasal wall increases the internal diameter of the nasal airway, thereby increasing dynamic nasal airflow. (*From* TerKonda RP, Sykes JM. Repairing the twisted nose. Otolaryngol Clin North Am 1999;32(1):61; with permission.)

More commonly, external valve insufficiency is a dynamic deformity caused by a weakened lateral nasal vestibular wall, exacerbated by trauma, which collapses on inspiration. Structures responsible include the upper and lower lateral cartilages and the fibrofatty tissue of the nasal ala. External nasal valve deformity may be a significant source of nasal airway obstruction in some patients. Constantian and Clardy[19] demonstrated that reconstruction of the external valve alone can improve total mean airflow by more than twice that of preoperative valves. Interestingly, this degree of airflow improvement is similar to that observed in patients in whom pure internal nasal valve dysfunction is corrected with dorsal or spreader grafts. Moreover, preliminary data for patients in whom both internal and external valve dysfunction are treated (without septal or turbinate surgery) reveal a mean threefold airflow increase, which suggests that the effects of internal and external valve reconstruction may be independent but not strictly additive, presumably because of valve interactions.[19]

Techniques used to address external valve collapse include alar batten grafting (as discussed in the previous section), lateral crural strut grafts, and, more recently, suturing of the lower lateral cartilage to the orbital rim.[13–15,19,20,26,27] Again, patients must be counseled that many of the techniques used to address nasal obstruction due to lateral wall or external valve collapse may change the appearance of the nose by widening it. First described in the mid-1990s, suture suspension of the upper and lower lateral cartilages to the inferior orbital rim has been used to stabilize the external valve against negative inspiratory forces and thereby improve nasal obstruction (**Fig. 8**).[26–30] In 2006, Most treated seven patients with external valve collapse with bone-anchored sutures and observed them for 32 to 390 days.[28] Average NOSE scores significantly decreased in these patients from 66.3 to 20.0 ($P < .01$).[28]

Caudal septal deviation is another cause of posttraumatic nasal obstruction in the lower third. When the displacement of the septum off the maxillary crest is responsible for the deflection and physical obstruction, it can be addressed by mobilizing the inferior and posterior aspect of the quadrangular cartilage and placing the septum back

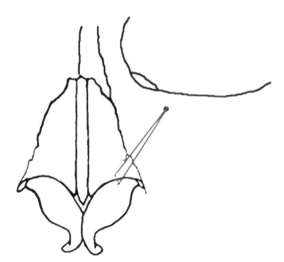

Fig. 8. Suture suspension of the upper and lower lateral cartilages to the inferior orbital rim has been used to stabilize the external valve against negative inspiratory forces. (*From* Roofe SB, Most SP. Placement of a lateral nasal suspension suture via an external rhinoplasty approach. Arch Facial Plast Surg 2007;9(3):215; with permission.)

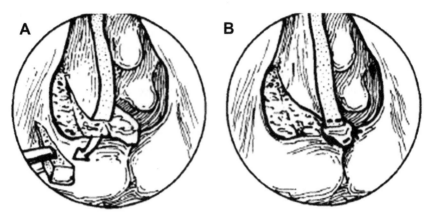

Fig. 9. When displacement of the septum off the maxillary crest is responsible for the deflection and physical obstruction, it can be addressed by mobilizing the inferior and posterior aspect of the quadrangular cartilage, resecting the inferior aspect of the nasal septum (A), and suture fixing the septum back into the midline (B). (From TerKonda RP, Sykes JM. Repairing the twisted nose. Otolaryngol Clin North Am 1999;32(1):59; with permission.)

into the midline (**Fig. 9**).[7] When severe anterior septal deviation is present, traditional septoplasty techniques are inadequate to effectively treat high septal or caudal septal deformities, especially without weakening tip support, further narrowing the internal nasal valve, or causing destabilization and saddling of the nasal dorsum. The technique of total removal, extracorporeal remodeling, and reimplantation of a severely deviated caudal septum was first published by King and Ashley in 1952.[29] This method has subsequently been modified over the last 50 years.[31–40] Most has demonstrated that anterior septal reconstruction, a more conservative approach to the traditional

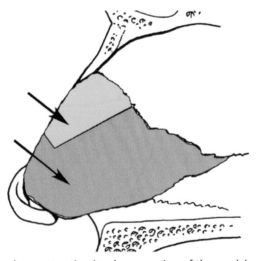

Fig. 10. Anterior septal reconstruction involves resection of the caudal septum (area in red) while preserving a dorsal strut, particularly at the keystone area (area in blue), the junction of the quadrangular cartilage to the bony septum and nasal bones. (From Most SP. Anterior septal reconstruction: outcomes after a modified extracorporeal septoplasty technique. Arch Facial Plast Surg 2006;8(3):203; with permission.)

extracorporeal septoplasty that preserves dorsal support, is effective in addressing nasal obstruction (**Fig. 10**). Average NOSE scores decreased significantly in patients who underwent anterior septal reconstruction with or without concomitant turbinate reduction, from 76.6 to 12.9 ($P < .01$).[34]

SUMMARY

The sequelae of trauma to the nose include nasal deformity and nasal obstruction that can have a long-term negative impact on patient quality of life and thus often require repair. Careful planning is critical to successful treatment of posttraumatic nasal obstruction. Dividing the nose into horizontal thirds assists in preoperative analysis and surgical treatment. Correcting nasal deformity and nasal obstruction are often conflicting objectives that are usually addressed simultaneously. Adequate treatment of posttraumatic nasal obstruction must address deflection of the bony nasal pyramid, septal deformities, especially caudal or dorsal, turbinate hypertrophy, and incompetence of both internal and external nasal valves.

REFERENCES

1. Rohrich RJ, Adams WP Jr. Nasal fracture management: minimizing secondary nasal deformities. Plast Reconstr Surg 2000;106(2):266–73.
2. Higuera S, Lee EI, Cole P, et al. Nasal trauma and the deviated nose. Plast Reconstr Surg 2007;120(7 Suppl 2):64S–75S.
3. Muraoka M, Nakai Y. Twenty years of statistics and observation of facial bone fracture. Acta Otolaryngol Suppl 1998;538:261–5.
4. Holt GR. Biomechanics of nasal septal trauma. Otolaryngol Clin North Am 1999; 32(4):615–9.
5. Murray JA, Maran AG, Mackenzie IJ, et al. Open vs closed reduction of the fractured nose. Arch Otolaryngol 1984;110(12):797–802.
6. Ramirez OM, Pozner JN. The severely twisted nose. Clin Plast Surg 1996;23: 327–40.
7. TerKonda RP, Sykes JM. Repairing the twisted nose. Otolaryngol Clin North Am 1999;32(1):53–64.
8. Verwoerd CDA, Verwoerd-Verhoef HL. Developmental aspects of the deviated nose. Facial Plast Surg 1989;6(2):95–100.
9. Lanfranchi PV, Steiger J, Soprano A, et al. Diagnostic and surgical endoscopy in functional rhinoplasty. Facial Plast Surg 2004;20:207–15.
10. Most SP. Trends in functional rhinoplasty. Arch Facial Plast Surg 2008;10(6): 410–3.
11. Most SP, Murakami CS. A modern approach to nasal osteotomies. Facial Plast Surg Clin North Am 2005;13(1):85–92.
12. Kim DW, Toriumi DM. Management of posttraumatic nasal deformities: the crooked nose and the saddle nose. Facial Plast Surg Clin North Am 2004; 12(1):111–32.
13. Park SS. Treatment of the internal nasal valve. Facial Plast Surg Clin North Am 1999;7:333–45.
14. Rohrich RJ, Hollier LH. Use of spreader grafts in the external approach to rhinoplasty. Clin Plast Surg 1996;23:255–62.
15. Sheen JH. Spreader graft: a method of reconstructing the roof of the middle nasal vault following rhinoplasty. Plast Reconstr Surg 1984;73:230–9.
16. Sancho BV, Molina AR. Use of septal cartilage homografts in rhinoplasty. Aesthetic Plast Surg 2000;24:357–63.

17. Romo T 3rd, Sclafani AP, Jacono AA. Nasal reconstruction using porous polyethylene implants. Facial Plast Surg 2000;16:55–61.
18. Schlosser RJ, Park SS. Surgery for the dysfunctional nasal valve. Arch Facial Plast Surg 1999;1:105–10.
19. Constantian MB, Clardy RB. The relative importance of septal and nasal valvular surgery in correcting airway obstruction in primary and secondary rhinoplasty. Plast Reconstr Surg 1996;98(1):38–54.
20. Andre R, Paun S, Viyk H. Endonasal spreader graft placement as treatment for internal nasal valve insufficiency. Arch Facial Plast Surg 2004;6(1):36–40.
21. Byrd HS, Meade RA, Gonyon DL Jr. Using the autospreader flap in primary rhinoplasty. Plast Reconstr Surg 2007;119(6):1897–902.
22. Alsarraf R, Murakami CS. The saddle nose deformity. Facial Plast Surg Clin North Am 1999;7:303–10.
23. Park SS. The flaring suture to augment the repair of the dysfunctional nasal valve. Plast Reconstr Surg 1998;101:1120–2.
24. Toriumi DM, Josen J, Weinberger M, et al. Use of alar batten grafts for correction of nasal valve collapse. Arch Otolaryngol Head Neck Surg 1997;123(8):802–8.
25. Egan KK, Kim DW. A novel intranasal stent for functional rhinoplasty and nostril stenosis. Laryngoscope 2005;115:903–9.
26. Roofe SB, Most SP. Placement of a lateral nasal suspension suture via an external rhinoplasty approach. Arch Facial Plast Surg 2007;9(3):214–6.
27. Wittkopf M, Wittkopf J, Ries WR. The diagnosis and treatment of nasal valve collapse. Curr Opin Otolaryngol Head Neck Surg 2008;16(1):10–3.
28. Most SP. Analysis of outcomes after functional rhinoplasty using a disease-specific quality-of-life instrument. Arch Facial Plast Surg 2006;8:306–9.
29. Paniello RC. Nasal valve suspension: an effective treatment for nasal valve collapse. Arch Otolaryngol Head Neck Surg 1996;122:1342–6.
30. King ED, Ashley FL. The correction of the internally and externally deviated nose. Plast Reconstr Surg 1952;10(2):116–20.
31. Gubisch W. The extracorporeal septum plasty: a technique to correct difficult nasal deformities. Plast Reconstr Surg 1995;95(4):672–82.
32. Gubisch W. Extracorporeal septoplasty for the markedly deviated septum. Arch Facial Plast Surg 2005;7(4):218–26.
33. Most SP. Anterior septal reconstruction: outcomes after a modified extracorporeal septoplasty technique. Arch Facial Plast Surg 2006;8(3):202–7.
34. Gerlinger I, Kárász T, Somogyvári K, et al. Extracorporal septal reconstruction with polydioxanone foil. Clin Otolaryngol 2007;32(6):465–70.
35. Illum P, Kristensen S, Jorgensen K, et al. Role of fixation in the treatment of nasal fractures. Clin Otolaryngol 1983;8(3):191–5.
36. Murakami CS, Bloom DC, Most SP. Managing the persistently crooked nose. In: Becker DG, Park SS, editors. Revision rhinoplasty. 1st edition. New York: Thieme Medical Publishers; 2008. p. 85–95.
37. Pontius AT, Leach JL Jr. New techniques for management of the crooked nose. Arch Facial Plast Surg 2004;6(4):263–6.
38. Rhee JS, Arganbright JM, McMullin BT, et al. Evidence supporting functional rhinoplasty or nasal valve repair: a 25-year systematic review. Otolaryngol Head Neck Surg 2008;139(1):10–20.
39. Roofe SB, Murakami CS. Treatment of the posttraumatic and postrhinoplasty crooked nose. Facial Plast Surg Clin North Am 2006;14(4):279–89.
40. Teichgraeber JF, Wainwright DJ. The treatment of nasal valve obstruction. Plast Reconstr Surg 1994;93:1174–82.

Treatment of Dorsal Deviation

Richard A. Zoumalan, MD[a,*], Michael A. Carron, MD[b],
Bobby A. Tajudeen[a], Philip J. Miller, MD[c]

KEYWORDS

• Rhinoplasty • Nasal • Deviation • Dorsal • Twisted • Nose

The deviated dorsum creates the appearance of a twisted, asymmetric, or deviated nose. This situation may create functional and aesthetic issues that require correction.[1,2] Correction of the dorsal deviation may present itself as a challenge to the rhinoplasty surgeon. The dorsum is a complex three-dimensional structure in which correcting a functional issue may have an impact on cosmesis and cosmetic correction may impair nasal function. Therefore, any attempt at straightening a dorsum should strive to maximize cosmetic outcome and maintain or improve nasal function. This can be a difficult task for the surgeon.

A proper skeletal support is necessary to provide long-term aesthetic and functional results. In the past, rhinoplasty was typically a reductive operation commonly resulting in loss of support, whereas the modern operation is focused on restructuring the nose.[3,4] To give the nose an appearance of being straight, the existing architecture is realigned or grafts are used to provide a symmetric and straight appearance. Most often, both strategies are used to achieve a straight and symmetric nose. Overall, autogenous cartilage is the material most commonly used to restructure the nose and provides material with which to strengthen, augment, camouflage, and reposition the deviated dorsum. Sources of autogenous cartilage are the nasal septum, auricular conchal cartilage, and costal cartilage.[5–7]

PATIENT ASSESSMENT

Deviations range from a subtle "C"-shaped deformity to a severe twisted nose deformity. Systematic facial analysis and evaluation of the dorsum are critical to correcting

[a] Department of Otolaryngology-Head and Neck Surgery, New York University School of Medicine, 550 First Avenue, NBV 5E5, New York, NY 10003, USA
[b] Facial Plastic and Reconstructive Surgery, Department of Otolaryngology-Head and Neck Surgery, Wayne State University School of Medicine, 4201 St. Antoine, 5E-UHC, Detroit, MI 48201, USA
[c] Department of Otolaryngology-Head and Neck Surgery, Division of Facial Plastic and Reconstructive Surgery, New York University School of Medicine, 60 East 56th, Third Floor, New York, NY 10022, USA
* Corresponding author.
E-mail address: richard.zoumalan@nyumc.org (R.A. Zoumalan).

Otolaryngol Clin N Am 42 (2009) 579–586
doi:10.1016/j.otc.2009.04.012
0030-6665/09/$ – see front matter © 2009 Elsevier Inc. All rights reserved.
oto.theclinics.com

a deformity of this type. Such an analysis is complicated by the fact that most faces, on close examination, are vertically or horizontally asymmetric. As such, aligning the nose perfectly with one side or half of the face may not make it symmetric with respect to the other side. For example, the inferior third of the face may not lie in direct midline alignment with the upper third of the face. Hence, making a dorsum that bisects those two midline points results in a nose angled to one side. These imperfections and asymmetries should be pointed out to the patient before any surgery.

Perhaps the only consistent reference point for an frontal or anterior-posterior (A-P) photograph is the center point between the medial canthi on the nose with the head in the Frankfort plane. The other facial landmarks tend to be ineffective for analysis of dorsal symmetry because of facial asymmetries.[8] A straight line is drawn from pupil to pupil. The center point between the medial canthi is marked. From this point, a straight midline vertical line is dropped intersecting the glabella, nasal dorsum, tip, columellar base, nasal spine, philtrum, upper incisors, and menton.[9] **Fig. 1** shows a patient with a very minimal upper third nasal deviation. In such cases where the deviation is subtle/minimal, a vertical line dropped from the centerpoint between the medial canthi or pupils can more clearly show this. Additionally, the rhinoplasty surgeon should analyze the patient's brow-aesthetic line on the A-P photograph. The nasal width should provide a graceful curvilinear line from brow to nasal tip. Deviation of the dorsum alters the brow-tip aesthetic and affects the contour of this line.[10] **Fig. 2** shows an appropriate brow-tip aesthetic line for a patient with a straight nose.

The upper, middle, and lower thirds of the dorsum are each analyzed independently and then together as a whole.[11,12] The upper third is composed of the nasal bones and the ascending process of the maxilla. The middle third is composed of the dorsal septum fused in the midline to the paired upper lateral cartilages. The lower third is the nasal tip, which includes the lower lateral cartilages, caudal septum, and alar base. Each third is recorded as being deviated to the left or right. It is clinically significant whether the upper, middle, or lower third is deviated because the surgical management of each third of the vault has its own set of maneuvers to straighten it.

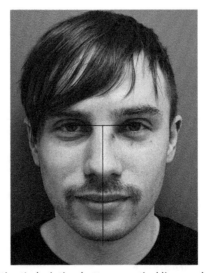

Fig. 1. To appreciate a patient's deviation better, a vertical line can be drawn from the center point between the pupils or medial canthi.

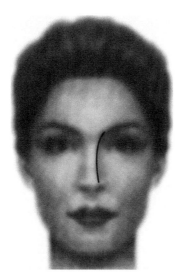

Fig. 2. Brow-tip aesthetic line.

In this article, the surgical approach to the deviated nose is based on this principle of thirds. **Fig. 3**A, B shows a patient with dorsal deviation to the left. The upper third (nasal bones) is not deviated. The middle and lower thirds of the nose are deviated to the right, however. **Fig. 3**C, D shows the patient after surgical straightening of the nose. These photographs were taken 6 months after surgery.

Integral to patient assessment is the assessment of the intended surgical approach. The approach for management of the deviated dorsum can be external or endonasal. The choice of approach used depends on the severity of the deviation and comfort level of the surgeon. The authors find that most maneuvers targeting the deviated nose can be comfortably performed with either approach. In the 1970s, Goodman and Charles[12] introduced a columellar incision to provide unparalleled exposure and facilitate open rhinoplasty as a means to preserve anatomic structure. This dramatically decreased the learning curve of surgeons attempting to perform a complex procedure. Yet, this comes at the expense of potentially increased operative time, prolonged postoperative swelling, scar contracture, and loss of nasal tip support. There is also the issue of an external scar that may heal conspicuously depending on a variety of factors. The advantages of endonasal rhinoplasty include decreased operative time, rapid recovery, and less significant scar contracture. These benefits come at a cost of a more limited exposure, however.[13]

MANAGEMENT OF THE UPPER THIRD

Treatment of the deviated upper third is tailored to the upper third deformity. The nasal bones as a unit may be twisted to the side, but the ascending processes of the maxilla are uninvolved. There may be a fracture (rare) of the entire bony complex unit to one side. More commonly, there are variations on those extremes. The treatment is osteotomies, and the specific osteotomy is based on the identified abnormality.

Deviation of the bony pyramid is corrected with osteotomies made at specific locations along the vertical plane of the bones, depending on the location of bony deviation. Once the bony dorsum is mobilized, it may be manipulated and straightened, and occasionally stented. Osteotomies may be performed in a variety of ways. They can be

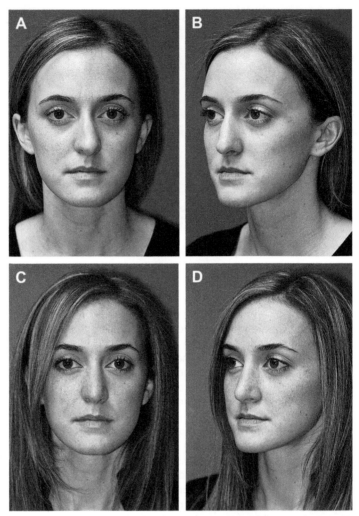

Fig. 3. (A, B) Dorsal deviation of the middle and lower thirds to the left. The upper third is relatively straight. (C, D) Six months after surgical correction of the deviation.

performed using a continuous technique, which is the most common method used. In this type of osteotomy, the cuts are made in a continuous fashion, through the nasal sidewall. Osteotomies can also be performed in a perforating fashion, which is a postage stamp type of sequential fracture using a narrow osteotome (2–3 mm). Osteotomies can also be performed by means of percutaneous perforations, which are also performed with a narrow osteotome. The type of osteotomy is insignificant as long as there is a cut through the bone that allows sufficient bone movement for the bony pyramid to be shifted to midline. Lateral osteotomies are ideally performed in a high-low-high fashion. The initial part of the osteotomy begins at the pyriform aperture (high point) and travels laterally toward the ipsilateral eye. As the osteotomy nears the nasal process of the maxilla (low point), it travels cephalically and medially toward a point just medial to the medial canthus (high point).

Medial osteotomies are performed in addition to lateral (occasionally intermediate) osteotomies to allow increased mobility before manipulation of the bones. A combination of osteotomies is usually sufficient to bring the bones back to midline; however, lateral osteotomies alone may suffice. Medial osteotomies are performed by making osteotomies that begin just lateral to the septal insertion into the underside of the nasal bones. These osteotomies are aimed laterally to avoid rocker deformity.

Dorsal hump reduction may obviate the need for medial osteotomies. This is determined by how much hump is removed. When an open roof deformity is created after significant hump reduction, lateral osteotomies alone suffice because the central portion of the bony pyramid is absent. Because the bone is removed from the osteotomy, there is no central bone available to cut with an osteotome. If dorsal hump reduction does not remove a significant portion of the bony roof, greenstick fracture may result if lateral osteotomies alone are performed because there remains a bony bridge from the end of the lateral osteotomy to the root of the nose. Greenstick fractures are not ideal because they maintain a spring-like tendency, resulting in a return of the bony pyramid to its original configuration in the postoperative period.[14]

Unilateral osteotomies can be performed in certain situations. The surgeon must be open to ways to reshape the upper third, including not only unilateral osteotomy but outfracture of nasal bones after osteotomy. The usual strategy of the facial plastic surgeon is to infracture nasal bones before trying to realign the nasal vault. In certain circumstances of severe deviation attributable to fracture, however, the pyramid is so deviated that a portion of bone must be outfractured.

In severe cases of deviation, a cross-root (or transverse-root) osteotomy can be performed. In this maneuver, a 2-mm osteotome can be used to make perforated percutaneous osteotomies in a horizontal fashion across the nasion, or just inferior to the nasal root. This series of perforations should connect the most cephalic aspect of the lateral osteotomies. This maneuver should provide tremendous mobility when combined with medial and lateral osteotomies. The bony dorsum can then be manipulated and molded with the opposite hand into place. This maneuver is usually used when medial and lateral osteotomies are insufficient in providing the mobility required for straightening.

MANAGEMENT OF THE MIDDLE THIRD

Straightening the middle third of a deviated dorsum can prove quite challenging. Minor concavities of the middle third can be addressed with onlay cartilage grafts placed in precise pockets or directly sutured onto the depression using an external rhinoplasty approach. Such onlay grafts do not improve nasal function and airflow, however, but are primarily for cosmetic improvement.[15] Management of a more severely deviated middle third requires more aggressive maneuvers to straighten the septum and the paired upper lateral cartilages to which it is fused in the midline.[16,17] Reorientation of the middle third should be performed subsequent to osteotomies so that the nose does not shift back toward the deviated position.

Integral to the management of middle third deviation is straightening the dorsal septum. This can be done in several ways. Septoplasty alone may be all that is needed and can be performed by means of a Killian, transfixion, hemitransfixion, or external rhinoplasty technique. Severe deviations sometimes require that the upper lateral cartilages be detached from the septum by means of an external rhinoplasty approach with open septal reconstruction. This view delivers unparalleled septal exposure, allowing for a more complicated and involved operation to straighten or replace the septum if need be.

The septum can be scored on its concave surface to help release the spring and allow it to be straightened. Scoring is not effective unless there is some type of dorsal and caudal support allowing the septum to stay in position after scoring. The cartilage still has some memory and strength, causing it to return to its original position. Portions of cartilage can be removed, but care must be taken to preserve 8 to 10 mm of dorsal and caudal septum to prevent saddle deformity attributable to septal weakening and collapse.

The spreader graft has become the "workhorse" graft for straightening of the middle third. Sheen[17] conceived the spreader graft a means of improving the transition between bone and cartilage and opening the internal nasal valve. This graft is placed in a pocket between the dorsal septum and the upper lateral cartilages. Spreader grafts can act to address concavities by augmenting the concave size.[14] They can also address the deviated dorsal septum by acting as a splint.

Spreader grafts are perhaps the most difficult of all grafts to be placed by means of an endonasal approach. Although the open approach facilitates an easier insertion, an endonasal approach is used by the senior author (PJM) in many instances. In cases of airway obstruction, the endonasal approach is ideal for placement of the graft. The submucosal placement offers the maximal opening of the internal nasal valve. A precise pocket is created along the lateral dorsum between the dorsal septum and upper lateral cartilages. A small freer is used to elevate the small pocket. If placed correctly, the graft should push the upper lateral cartilage laterally. Suture placement is not required if the pocket is precise.

In a severely deviated middle third, disarticulation of the upper lateral cartilages may be necessary because of traumatic upper lateral cartilage avulsions. It may also help to visualize the deviated dorsal septum. In this instance, the placement of the spreader graft is best placed extramucosally. This can be challenging using an endonasal technique. A converse retractor is used to elevate the soft tissues over the dorsum. The upper lateral cartilage is disarticulated from the nasal septum with careful effort to stay extramucosal. The fashioned spreader graft is placed in the pocket and sutured with 4–0 polydioxanone (PDS) suture.

In patients with severe deviation or fracture that cannot be effectively straightened using grafts and scoring, reconstruction of a large portion of the septal structure may be performed. Subtotal reconstruction of the cartilaginous dorsum is an effective tool for severe septal deviation or fracture not amenable to scoring or cartilaginous reinforcement. This procedure requires an open approach and a large piece of cartilage for harvest. If this is not available, auricular or costal cartilage harvest is recommended.

The authors prefer to use autogenous cartilage for restructuring and reinforcing the nasal septum. The three options for autogenous cartilage are nasal septum, auricular cartilage, and costal cartilage. The authors prefer to use nasal septal cartilage because of ease of harvest and use. If septal cartilage is not available or is insufficient, conchal cartilage can be a good graft site. At times, however, there is not sufficient cartilage from the septum or ear or the cartilage is not sturdy enough for the needs of the patient. In this case, costal cartilage is harvested.

RELATION OF THE LOWER THIRD

Septal deviation may not only cause dorsal deviation but nasal obstruction by its intrusion on the normal airway. Deviation of the lower third is most commonly attributable to caudal septal deflection. The caudal septum is a critical structure providing support to the tip of the nose. Because the septum is situated between the lower lateral cartilages in the midline, deviation of it has a tendency to deviate the lower third dorsum to the right or the left.

Mild caudal septal deflections may be treated with a "swinging door" technique. In this maneuver, the caudal septum is freed down to the maxillary spine, "flipped" to the other side of the spine, and sutured to periosteum to fix it. Normally, a pocket is created between the medial crura to accommodate the caudal septum in its new position. If necessary, a small margin of caudal septum is excised at its inferior margin to permit its "swing" to the contralateral side of the nasal spine. The concave side of the septum can be scored to straighten it and to decrease its tendency to "spring back" into its previous position as a result of memory of the cartilage. In more severe cases, the caudal septum may need a more complex correction with removal and replacement with autogenous cartilage from the auricle or rib. This septal graft is then secured to the remnant of the quadrangular cartilage, the anterior nasal spine, and between the lower lateral cartilages.

SUMMARY

The deviated nose is a complex problem with a variety of solutions. A simple approach for the deviated dorsum with surgical relevance is thinking of the nose as being divided into thirds. Tailoring maneuvers to alleviate problems in each specific third helps the surgeon deal with deviations in an effective and straightforward manner.

REFERENCES

1. Johnson CM Jr, Anderson JR. The deviated nose—its correction. Laryngoscope 1977;87(10 Pt 1):1680–4.
2. Gunther JP, Rorich RJ. Management of the deviated nose. The importance of septal reconstruction. Clin Plast Surg 1988;15(1):43–55.
3. Papel ID, Larrabee W, Holt G, et al. Rhinoplasty. In: Papel I, editor. Facial plastic and reconstructive surgery. 2nd edition. New York: Thieme Publishing; 2000. p. 205–8.
4. Tardy ME, Toriumi DM. Philosophy and principles of rhinoplasty. In: Papel LE, Nachlas NE, editors. Facial plastic and reconstructive surgery. New York: Thieme Publishing; 2000. p. 278–94.
5. Gunter JP, Friedman RM. Lateral crural strut graft: technique and clinical applications in rhinoplasty. Plast Reconstr Surg 1997;99(4):943–52 [discussion: 953–5].
6. Toriumi DM, Josen J, Weinberger M, et al. Use of alar batten grafts for correction of nasal valve collapse. Arch Otolaryngol Head Neck Surg 1997;123(8):802–8.
7. Tardy ME Jr, Becker D, Weinberger M. Illusions in rhinoplasty. Facial Plast Surg 1995;11(3):117–37.
8. Farkus LG. Asymmetry of the head and face. In: Farkus LG, editor. Anthropometry of the head and face. 2nd edition. New York: Raven Press; 1981. p. 102–11.
9. Vuyk HD. A review of practical guidelines for correction of the deviated, asymmetric nose. Rhinology 2000;38(2):72–8.
10. Powell N, Humphreys B. Proportions of the aesthetic face. New York: Thieme Stratton, Inc; 1984. p. 110–105.
11. Murakami CS, Larrabee WF. Comparison of osteotomy techniques in the treatment of nasal fractures. Facial Plast Surg 1992;8(4):209–19.
12. Goodman WS, Charles DA. Technique of external rhinoplasty. J Otolaryngol 1978; 7:13–7.
13. Shah AR, Miller PJ. Structural approach to endonasal rhinoplasty. Facial Plast Surg. 2006;22(1):55–60.

14. Toriumi D, Ries W. Innovative surgical management of the crooked nose. Facial Plast Surg Clin North Am 1993;1:63–78.
15. Constantian M. An algorithm for correction of the asymmetric nose. Plast Reconstr Surg 1984;83:801–3.
16. Anderson J. Straightening the crooked nose. Trans Am Acad Ophthalmol Otolaryngol 1972;76:938–45.
17. Sheen JH. Spreader graft: a method of reconstructing the roof of the middle nasal vault following rhinoplasty. Plast Reconstr Surg 1984;73:230–9.

Index

Note: Page numbers of article titles are in **boldface** type.

A

Abscess, septal, following septoplasty, 469–471
Adhesions, as complication of septoplasty, 474–475
Airway blockage, due to enlargement of middle turbinates, 559, 562
Alar batten grafts, for deformities of middle third of nose, 572–573, 574
    for external nasal valves, 504–508
Alar strut grafts, for external nasal valves, 508–509
Alloplasts, for nasal augmentation, 443–445
Anesthesia, for septoplasty, complications of, 464–465
Autografts, for nasal augmentation, 445–447, 449

B

Batten grafting, in caudal nasal septum deviation, 432–433
Brow-tip aesthetic line, 580, 581
Butterfly grafts, in dysfunction of nasal valves, 501

C

Cartilage(s), costal, nasal reconstruction of leprosy nose using, **547–555**
    reconstruction of, in reconstruction of caudal nasal septum, 434
    lower lateral, cephalic malposition of, 542–543, 545
        airflow obstruction in, 543
        cosmetic and functional effects of, **539–546**
        cosmetic deformity in, 543
        rhinoplasty in, endonasal approach for, 539–541, 542, 544–545
            nasal evaluation for, 543–544
            open approach for, 544
    reshaping of, in deviation of caudal nasal septum, 430–433
    suture suspension of, for treatment of deformities of lower third of nose, 575
Cartilage graft, striated septal, in dysfunction of nasal valves, 501, 503
Cerebrospinal fluid leak, due to septoplasty, 466–468
Columella, retraction of, following septoplasty, 478–479
Cosmetic deformities, in cephalic malposition of lower lateral cartilages, **539–546**
Costal cartilage, reconstruction of, in reconstruction of caudal nasal septum, 434
Crura, paradoxical lateral, external nasal valves and, 508–509

D

Dorsal inlay, with septoplasty, to correct "saddling," 535, 536
Dorsal onlay grafts, for treatment of deformities of middle third of nose, 572

Otolaryngol Clin N Am 42 (2009) 587–592
doi:10.1016/S0030-6665(09)00080-2
0030-6665/09/$ – see front matter © 2009 Elsevier Inc. All rights reserved.

Dorsum, deviated, patient assessment in, 579–581
    treatment of, **579–586**
    lower third of, 580, 584–585
    middle third of, 580
        management of, 583
    upper third of, 580
        management of, 580

E

Endonasal approach, for surgical management of septal perforation, 487
Endoscopy, for assessment of nasal obstruction, 561–562
    for septoplasty, 563
    to assess septal perforation, 484

F

Flaring sutures ("Park sutures"), for treatment of deformities of middle third of nose, 572
    in dysfunction of nasal valves, 500–501
Free flap, radial forearm, in surgical management of septal perforation, 491

H

Hematoma, septal, following septoplasty, 469–471
Hemorrhage, as result of septoplasty, 465–466
Holoprosencephaly, 523–524
Homografts, for nasal augmentation, 447–450

I

Incisor, maxillary, single, and congenital stenosis of nasal pyriform aperture, 523–524
Infection, following septoplasty, 468–469

L

Leprosy, drug regimen in, 550
    epidemiology of, 549–550
    incidence of, 547
    saddle-nose deformity in, correction of, 551
        severe, augmentation for, 551–554
Leprosy nose, nasal reconstruction of, using costal cartilage, **547–555**
        case report of, 548, 549–550, 551, 552, 553

M

Monarch adjustable implant, in dysfunction of nasal valves, 503
Mucosal flap, tunneled sublabial, in surgical management of septal perforation, 491

N

Nasal base, widened, following septoplasty, 477–478
Nasal congestion, medical management of, 429
    surgical management of, 430

Nasal obstruction, and nasal deformity, endonasal rhinoplasty in, case illustrating, 539–541, 542
    causes of, in case report of aesthetic revision rhinoplasty, 562–563
    correction of, aesthetic revision rhinoplasty and, **557–565**
        case report of, 557–558
    differential diagnosis of, 558, 560
    endoscopic examination of, 561–562
    history of, and physical examination in, 558–561
    imaging of, 561
    in chronic sinusitis, 563
    in deformities of caudal and dorsal nasal septum, 528
    in deviated caudal nasal septum, 427
    in deviation of nasal septum, 562–563
    posttraumatic, treatment of caudal septal deviation in, 575–579
    septoplasty in, 427–428
    treatment of, in posttraumatic nose, **567–578**
Nasal septal button, in septal perforation, 486
Nasal septum, anatomy of, 513–514
    caudal, anatomy of, 428–429
        deviation of, **427–436**
            aesthetic problems in, 427
            batten grafting in, 432–433
            cartilage reshaping in, 430–433
            classification of, 430
            extracorporeal resection in, 433–434
            nasal obstruction in, 427
            septal reconstruction in, 433–434
            septal repositioning in, 430
            spreader grafts in, 430–431, 435
            suture technique in, 431
            tongue-in-groove technique in, 431, 432
            treatment of, in posttraumatic nasal obstruction, 575–579
            wedging, scoring, and morselizing in, 431
        reconstruction of, costal cartilage reconstruction in, 434
            in cartilage depleted nose, 434–435
            polydioxanone foil in, 434
    caudal and dorsal, deformities of, nasal obstruction in, 528
    deformities of, history of correction of, 429
    deviations of, diagnosis of, 515–516
        indications and applications of open septoplasty in, 517–518
        nasal obstruction in, 562–563
    dorsal, deviated, open septoplasty in, 517
        deviations of, septoplasty in, 530–532
    overcorrected, septoplasty and, 471, 472
    perforation of. See Septal perforation.
    physiology of, 514–515
    reconstruction of, caudal nasal septum deviation, 433–434
    short, open septoplasty in, 517
    suturing of, in septoplasty, 534–536
Nasal valve(s), anatomy of, 495–496
    classification of, 496

Nasal (*continued*)
    collapse of, evaluation of, 563
    dysfunction of, butterfly grafts in, 501
        etiologies of, 496–497
        flaring sutures ("Park sutures") in, 500–501
        intranasal Z-plasty in, 503
        Monarch adjustable implant in, 503
        patient evaluation in, 497–498
        splay graft in, 502–503
        spreader grafts in, 499–500, 501, 502
        striated septal cartilage graft in, 501, 503
        surgical treatments of, 498–503
    external, alar batten grafts for, 504–508
        alar strut grafts for, 505, 506–507, 508
        paradoxical lateral crura and, 508–509
        surgical management of, 504–509
    management of, in septoplasty, 530–532
    obstruction of, nonsurgical treatments of, 498
    physiology of, 496
    surgical and nonsurgical treatments of, **495–511**
Nose, cartilage-depleted, reconstruction of caudal nasal septum in, 434–435
    deformity of, and nasal obstruction, endonasal rhinoplasty in, case illustrating, 539–541, 542
    leprous, nasal reconstruction of, using costal cartilage, **547–555**
    lower third of, treatment of deformities of, in posttraumatic obstruction, 574–577
    middle third of, treatment of deformities of, in posttraumatic obstruction, 570–573, 574
    posttraumatic, analysis of, 568–569
        treatment of nasal obstruction in, **567–578**
    structural support of, 437–438
    trauma to, etiology of, 567
    upper third of, treatment of deformities of, in posttraumatic obstruction, 569–570, 571

P

Pedicled flap, inferior turbinate, in surgical management of septal perforation, 490–491
Polydioxanone foil, in reconstruction of caudal nasal septum, 434
Pyriform aperture, nasal, anatomy and embryology of, 521–522
        congenital stenosis of, **521–525**
            and single maxillary incisor, 523–524
            treatment and management of, 524
        evaluation of, 522–524
        sublabial approach to, 522

R

Rhinoplasty, aesthetic revision, and causes of nasal obstruction in, case report of, 562–563
        and correction of nasal obstruction, **557–565**
            case report of, 557–558
    endonasal approach for, in cephalic malposition of lower lateral cartilages, 539–541, 542, 544–545
    external, as approach for surgical management of septal perforation, 490–491

functional, outcomes of, 509–510
nasal evaluation for, in cephalic malposition of lower lateral cartilages, 543–544
open approach for, in cephalic malposition of lower lateral cartilages, 544

S

Saddle nose deformity, catastrophic-major reconstruction (type V), 442, 446
     reconstruction of, 456–458
    classification and treatment of, **437–461**
    classification of, 439–442
    definition of, 438, 439
    due to septoplasty, 477
    etiology of, 438
    in leprosy, correction of, 551
    major-composite recontruction (type III), 440, 444
     reconstruction of, 453–456
    minor-cosmetic concealment (type I), 440, 442
     reconstruction of, 450–451
    moderate-cartilage vault restoration (type II), 440, 443
     reconstruction of, 451–553
    pseudosaddle (type 0), 440, 442
     reconstruction of, 450–451
    reconstructive materials for, 443–450
    reconstructive options in, 450–456
    severe, in leprosy, augmentation for, 551–554
    structural recontruction (type IV), 440–442, 445
     reconstruction of, 456
Sensory disturbances, following septoplasty, 475–476
Septal perforation, complications of, 483–484
    differential diagnosis of, 485
    endoscopy to assess, 484
    evaluation of, 484–485
    nasal hygiene in, 485–486
    nasal septal button in, 486
    nonsurgical treatment of, 485–486
    surgical management of, **483–493**
     aesthetic considerations for, 491–492
     endonasal approach for, 487
     external rhinoplasty approach for, 487–490
     facial artery musculomucosal flap for, 491
     inferior turbinate pedicle flap in, 490–491
     presurgical considerations for, 486–487
     radial forearm free flap in, 491
     tunneled sublabial mucosal flap in, 491
Septoplasty, adhesions or synechiae as complication of, 474–475
    anesthesia for, complications of, 464–465
    cerebrospinal fluid leak due to, 466–468
    columella retraction following, 478–479
    complications of, aesthetic, 476–479
     avoidance and management of, **463–481**
     functional, 465–476

Septoplasty (*continued*)
    deformities after, 476–477
    dorsal inlay with, to correct "saddling," 535, 536
    endoscopic, 563
    general approach for, 528–536
    hemorrhage as result of, 465–466
    history of, 527
    in dorsal septal deviations, 532–534
    in nasal obstruction, 427–428
    infection following, 468–469
    loss of tip projection following, 478
    management of nasal valve in, 528–530
    open, history of, 513
        indications and treatment using, **513–519**
        specific indications and applications of, 517
        technique of, 516–517
    overcorrected septum and, 471, 472
    pearls, **527–537**
    preoperative planning and evaluation for, 463–464
    saddle nose deformity due to, 477
    sensory disturbances following, 475–476
    septal hematoma or abscess following, 469–471
    septal perforation due to, 472–474
    septal suturing in, 534–536
    widened nasal base following, 477–478
Sinusitis, chronic, nasal obstruction in, 563
Splay graft, in dysfunction of nasal valves, 502–503
Spreader grafts, for treatment of deformities of middle third of nose, 572, 573, 574
    in dysfunction of nasal valves, 499–500, 501, 502
Submucous resection, in obstruction of nasal septum, 527
Suture suspension of cartilages, for treatment of deformities of lower third of nose, 575
Suture technique, caudal nasal septum deviation, 431
Sutures, flaring ("Park sutures"), in deformities of middle third of nose, 572
    in dysfunction of nasal valves, 500–501
Synechiae, as complication of septoplasty, 474–475

    T

Tip projection, loss of, following septoplasty, 478
Tongue-in-groove technique, in caudal nasal septum deviation, 431, 432
Trauma, to nose. See *Nose, posttraumatic*.
Turbinates, middle, enlargement of, airway blockage due to, 559, 562

    X

Xenographs, for interposition graft for nasal augmentation, 450

    Z

Z-plasty, intranasal, in dysfunction of nasal valves, 503

Moving?

Make sure your subscription moves with you!

To notify us of your new address, find your **Clinics Account Number** (located on your mailing label above your name), and contact customer service at:

E-mail: elspcs@elsevier.com

800-654-2452 (subscribers in the U.S. & Canada)
314-453-7041 (subscribers outside of the U.S. & Canada)

Fax number: 314-523-5170

Elsevier Periodicals Customer Service
11830 Westline Industrial Drive
St. Louis, MO 63146

*To ensure uninterrupted delivery of your subscription, please notify us at least 4 weeks in advance of move.

Printed and bound by CPI Group (UK) Ltd, Croydon, CR0 4YY

03/10/2024

01040463-0014